ADHD

A MODERN LEXICON

MERLIN GOLDMAN PhD

Miracle Fish

I'm totally wired...
My heart and I agree...
I'm always worried.

Totally Wired by The Fall

Synopsis

This book provides a short but informative overview of several common traits of ADHD. Over about two dozen chapters, *ADHD: A Modern Lexicon* discusses the many common features of ADHD using modern terminology. While some descriptors are well known, several are less so. Each is described with clarity and where possible, external, or personal examples are given. While not a self-help book, it does contain methods to counteract some of the more negative aspects of ADHD. All the ADHD-related terms are defined in the glossary.

Contents

INTRODUCTION

This book is intended to create a short introduction to **ADHD** using modern terminology. ADHD stands for attention deficit hyperactivity disorder although sometimes hyperactivity is dropped (**ADD**). For simplicity, I'll use ADHD throughout the book.

ADHD is used to describe a collection of symptoms that derive from a different brain structure. It's genetic and hereditary. Individuals with ADHD, who I'll refer to as **ADHDers**, don't get **dopamine** in quantities sufficient to maintain *normal* behaviour. This results in the symptoms or behaviours covered in this book, split into chapters, followed by a shorter section on things ADHDers dislike, and then a few methods that can be used to manage ADHD. And finally, some general tips and tricks.

ADHD was first discovered in the US by psychiatrist Charles Bradley in 1937 when he administered Benzedrine sulphate, an amphetamine, to children diagnosed with behavioural disorders. Bradley gave the children the stimulant for their headaches and by chance, it produced a calming effect, allowing them to concentrate. After a week, many of the patients were able to focus on their studies.[1] From then on, generations of children (and some adults) have been given **Ritalin**, along with several other versions of amphetamine. They're taken orally and come in different strengths with short and long-lasting formulations.

It's likely ADHD has been with us a long time. In 1904, *The Lancet* published a poem called *The Story of Fidgety Philip*. As long as there have been risk takers and wildly creative people, there have been people with ADHD. I will refer to some individuals by name. This is not meant to be diagnosis at a distance, but merely to give examples of well-known and visible individuals who demonstrate ADHD-like traits.

This book is not written from a medical perspective or as a how-to guide to live with ADHD. But I do give some tips. It's meant to provide a handy, short guide to understand some of the traits of ADHD, as experienced by me using colloquialisms. Since my diagnosis a few years ago, I've been able to catalogue the behaviours that I've identified as typical of someone with ADHD. This is mostly subjective, but the rest is based on my clinical diagnosis, academic

1 Madeleine P. Strohl. (2011) *Bradley's Benzedrine studies on children with behavioral disorders.* Yale J Biol Med. 2011 Mar; 84(1): 27–33.

reading, and specialist counselling. This book should appeal to those who believe they have ADHD or may have been recently diagnosed. It may also help to enlighten those who know someone with ADHD and want to learn more about it.

About 4% of the population have ADHD. This sits within a neurodivergent group, that includes other conditions like autism or dyspraxia, that accounts for about 15% of the population. In many Western countries, diagnosis at school is now relatively common. This usually reveals a parent with ADHD and often other family members. In recent years, there's been an upswell in adult diagnosis, in some cases triggered by the Covid-19 pandemic or greater awareness. In the UK, several celebrities, particularly comedians, have revealed they've been diagnosed.

People with ADHD are sometimes summarised as being creative, caring, and funny. From my experience, these are broadly true categorisations. This is not to say that someone without ADHD can't also be those things. It's just a short, positive summation. ADHDers also seem drawn to certain professions e.g. healthcare workers, e-sport gamers, entertainers, plumbers, electricians. They're also the ones that sends **memes**, don't do small talk, and are always busy and often late.

ADHDers are often risk takers – the person that thinks it's fun to climb a tree or jump from a plane. They're the person who stays up late then sleeps in. Or can't eat the same thing twice in a row. They're the soul of the party and the person who can't stop talking. They ask questions in classes they like but drift off in those that bore them. They love learning, trying new hobbies, or visiting new places. They can't sit still. Maybe this sounds like you?

Not every ADHDer behaves the same but I believe that many of the traits are common but vary in severity. Many adult ADHDers live successful lives, but some struggle, and can take some serious wrong turns. There are many factors at play here: the severity of their ADHD, their family or work environment, social life, medication, self-awareness about their condition or whether they've had a formal diagnosis.

Most of this book is based on personal observation but it does also include the results of research. Some of this is of the more academic type e.g. books, papers, articles but there's also plenty gleaned from YouTube, Instagram, or TikTok. The latter two have become an amusing source of short insights into ADHD.

Many with ADHD have developed methods to cope with the least debilitating aspects of it. For most, this has been a subconscious path of trial and error. Often ADHDers mask their natural behaviour and conform to social norms. Sometimes this can be straightforward e.g. engaging in social niceties. Or they overcompensate e.g. arriving very early for a meeting rather than being late. Does **masking** have negative consequences? Probably, although it's hard to quantify.

My experience of ADHD exists before and after my diagnosis. Pre-diagnosis, it wasn't overtly apparent to me or anyone else (unless they didn't want to say something). I could concentrate at school and was mostly non-disruptive. However, I enjoyed school and found most subjects interesting. And while I did tend to sit still, I could make cheeky comments and enjoyed practical jokes.

Since my diagnosis in 2021, I can reflect on my behaviour with a new perspective. I can see how it's impacted my life – in both positive and negative ways. And today, I can observe how it's affecting my behaviour in real time. For the most part, I try to work with it. I go with the flow, so to speak, rather than try to moderate it too much. For example, I might walk rather than get the bus, as this avoids both waiting for one, and gives me dopamine from the exercise.

Other times, I'll acknowledge that the path it's leading me down could be problematic and try to mitigate. For example, a recent passion of mine is synthesisers. I'm aware that there's a danger of spending large amounts of money on this new hobby, then losing interest. So, I buy second hand and have a price limit. I also know they can be sold (if I can manage the **admin**).

This book uses modern terminology while at the same time giving enough basic information, so even someone with no knowledge can read it from start to finish. I hope it provides some new insights into the condition along with a few tips to help manage it. I think the book can be read in several ways. If you know quite a bit about ADHD, skip the Some Basics section. If you're keen to learn about a specific trait, jump to it. I'll also provide some academic and other references as footnotes.

Above all, I hope you're at least entertained or informed by **ADHD: A Modern Lexicon**.

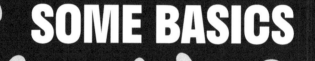

SOME BASICS

Diversity

It's quite clear we've come a long way in terms of diversity and representation. But there's still a large amount of ignorance about difference in all its forms: genetic, cultural, sexual. In this book, I'm focusing on the differences in brain type. Our current understanding is that there are both structural and neurochemical differences between those who are neurotypical (**NT**) and those who are neurodiverse (**ND**). The NT person is in the majority, and they've shaped society to their preferences and set the template for what it is to be *normal*.

The NT person has traits too. But these aren't ones we tend to focus on except in contrast to those who don't conform to them. The NT stereotype is someone who works nine to five, has a family, enjoys a pint in the pub with their mates at the weekend and goes on holiday in the summer.

Let's do some maths. At a rough approximation, there are one in 25 people with ADHD.[2] That's about 2.5 million people in the UK. It was thought that only about one in 100 have autism spectrum disorder (**ASD**). It's now thought that at least half of those diagnosed with ADHD also have ASD, and at least half of those with ASD have ADHD. Until quite recently, the discussion about neurodiversity has treated ADHD and ASD as separate conditions but things seem to be changing.[3]

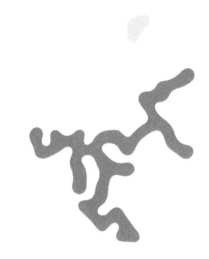

2 Vaziri-Harami R, Khademi M, Zolfaghari A, Vaziri-Harami S. (2024)
   *Patterns of substance use and initiation timing in adults with substance
   abuse: a comparison between those with and without attention deficit
   hyperactivity disorder.* Ann Med Surg (Lond). 2024 Jun 13; 86(8):4397-4401.
3 https://www.theguardian.com/lifeandstyle/2024/apr/04/audhd-what-is-
   behind-rocketing-rates-life-changing-diagnosis

SOME BASICS

Diagnosis

There are several ways to diagnose ADHD. Each has merits and drawbacks. Often the first route is an observation that they have traits like others diagnosed with ADHD or by someone commenting on their behaviour. While the latter might be gentler, both are a shock. For me, it was realising that I had many of the traits of a friend who'd recently been professionally diagnosed. I also went through a list of seventy-two traits someone with ADHD published online and found that I displayed most of them too.

For many, a self-diagnosis, although crude, is sufficient. An official confirmation is not something that they need or would be helpful. "I've survived this long with it, what more do I need to know?" But for others, a formal diagnosis might be reassuring and open other channels of support. In the UK, the first port of call is the **NHS** via a general practitioner (GP). At the end of the 2010s, waiting times for a formal diagnosis were in months. The Covid-19 pandemic unearthed many undiagnosed adults, extending waiting times to years.[4]

In England, the Right to Choose scheme provides a shortcut of sorts if you request a diagnosis via Psychiatry UK. It provides a streamlined process that reduces the waiting times. This consists of answering some written questions and at least one face-to-face meeting. The process is efficient but high level and can be disappointing.

For myself, I chose to see a private doctor who specialised in neurodivergence (and had ADHD themselves) who offered a speedier diagnosis. I had to complete a few questionnaires, an online test and two video calls. The documents I completed were:

The *Barkley Adult ADHD Rating Scale–IV (BAARS-IV)* (Guilford Press, 2011). This asks the subject to assess their behaviour within four categories: inattention, hyperactivity, impulsivity, and sluggish cognitive tempo.

4 https://www.additudemag.com/adhd-symptoms-diagnosed-treated-in-pandemic

A series of questions related to historical data in the areas: medical, family, developmental, education, work, and relationships.

The *Wender-Utah Rating Scale (WURS-25)*. I completed an abbreviated version of this document that asked questions related to my experience as a child.

The Hospital Anxiety and Depression Scale (Zigmond and Snaith, Acta Psychiatrica Scandinavica, 1983). The questions relate mostly to the frequency at which feelings occur e.g. panic, cheerfulness.

The *autism-spectrum quotient (AQ)* (Baron-Cohen, Wheelwright, Skinner, Martin, and Clubley, 2001). This is a questionnaire used to assess the subject's autism-spectrum quotient.

I also completed the *QbCheck* test provided by Qbtech. This can be completed at home and measures the three core symptoms of ADHD. It takes about twenty minutes and provides an objective measure. It gives you plenty of raw data in terms of how you performed during the test along with a score suggesting the extent to which you present with ADHD symptoms. I was at the mild end of the scale. The total cost was under £1,000 and took about a month.

SOME BASICS

Disability

ADHD can be so severe, making daily life highly challenging, that it'll be defined as a disability and therefore covered by the Equality Act 2010. This legislation seeks to protect twelve characteristics, one of which is disability. A disability is defined as a physical or mental impairment that has a substantial and long-term adverse effect on a person's ability to carry out normal day-to-day activities. Therefore, there remains some interpretation on whether an individual would feel that they're disabled. I suspect many with mild ADHD would say they're not disabled. But it's a personal choice.

The Equality Act brings with it a duty to make adjustments so that any person with one of the twelve characteristics is not disadvantaged. For someone with ADHD, who believes they need support to study or work, a discussion with the appointed contact point can be beneficial. Sometimes simple adjustments are all that are needed. For me, I have someone who helps manage my meeting calendar.

In the UK, the Access to Work scheme provides a formal route for support. For someone with ADHD it can provide a grant to help pay for practical support with work. This includes:

- Specialist equipment.
- Mental health support.
- Support workers.

I found the online application process to be quick and quite straightforward, but I suspect my ADHD is not severe enough to qualify for much, if any, support.

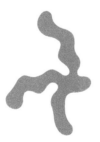

SOME BASICS

Dopamine

Dopamine or 3,4-dihydroxyphenethylamine is a neuromodulatory molecule synthesised in the brain and kidneys of most animals (and some plants). For our purposes, dopamine's key function is its role in *reward-motivated behaviour*. For the NT person, they receive dopamine from completing tasks, whether it be folding the laundry or taking out the rubbish (**motivational salience**). For the ADHDer, there's no dopamine reward unless it can be made interesting e.g. throwing the socks into the laundry basket. For most, completing a task gives the ADHDer a sense of *relief* rather than a feeling of *satisfaction*.

The ADHDer has decreased dopamine activity due to a reduced absorption caused by a faulty receptor. Dopamine receptors are thought to be involved in many neurological processes other than motivational salience. These include cognition, memory, learning, and fine motor control and likely contribute to many of the observed traits. For example, dopamine receptors control neural signalling involved in spatial working memory. Spatial memory is responsible for the recording of information needed to get somewhere or recall where you've left an object or a past event. I use a Sat Nav religiously, even to places I've been before. I forget where I've left objects so often, I have two of everything.

Before dopamine, norepinephrine was thought to be the key ADHD neurotransmitter, due to its role in regulating attention and alertness. Both now seem to be important, and many drugs target both. And the newest also increase levels of **serotonin**, involved in mood.

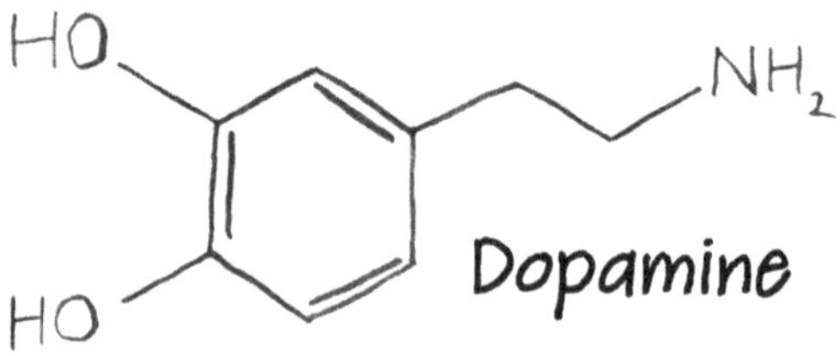

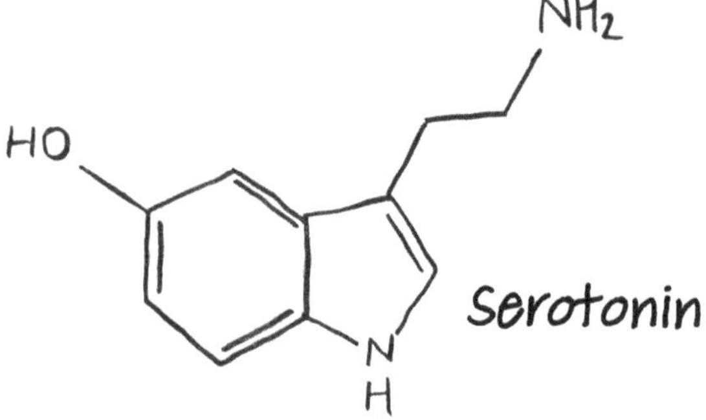

HO

NH$_2$

Dopamine

NH$_2$

HO

H
N

Serotonin

SOME BASICS

Severity

Whereas autism is a range of traits, ADHD is a more like a common set of features which every ADHDer has, but to a lesser or greater extent. It's more like a fuel gauge. Appropriately, the QbCheck test provides a score much like a fuel gauge. If green represents being NT, I slipped into the red. ADHD diagnoses are often classed as either mild, moderate, or severe. They will often also determine whether the patient is primarily inattentive, hyperactive-impulsive, or a combination.

The severity of one's ADHD is fundamental to an individual's ability to cope with 'normal' life. While even the most severely affected ADHDer may have found a way to live happily, a slight hiccup in their carefully or accidentally crafted world, can bring it all down very quickly. Someone with weaker ADHD symptoms, will probably cope. Awareness of where you are on the

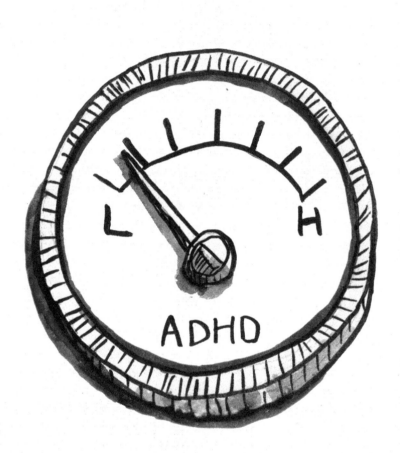

scale can help an ADHDer create a solid framework for successful living.

While this book's primary intention is not to provide a menu of coping mechanisms, some will be mentioned that have worked for me and others. Let's move on to the Behaviours section, which will catalogue the most common traits, using the most current terminology.

BEHAVIOURS

BEHAVIOURS

Bored

Many things in life are boring but for the ADHDer, some can be excruciating: waiting in queues, downloading files, or double maths (when you hate maths). Many times, I've given up standing in a queue for lunch, only to join another, and sometimes even another. If I'd stayed in the first one, I'd have been served first. But at the time that doesn't matter, if the queue's moving too slowly, I'm off. It's satisfying to have been decisive (even if I missed out on my preferred choice and ultimately the whole thing takes longer).

Each ADHDer will have different touch points. Long car journeys can be challenging due to their monotony. Anything more than one or two hours and I'll need a break. Repetition can be killer. My father would never drive the same way twice. We enjoyed plenty of scenic detours through London suburbs. I walk home from work a different way each day.

Perhaps the worst sort of boring, is having *nothing* to do. In these circumstances, the ADHDer might be able to grab dopamine through one of their preferred methods. Playing a game or **doomscrolling** on my phone is a simple solution to a slow queue. Doodling helps me to manage an unengaging talk or meeting. Sometimes, only a more extreme approach will work. I'm reminded of the scenes in the film *Aftersun*[5] when Calum goes for a midnight swim or when Julie gate-crashes a party in *The Worst Person in the World*.[6] In these moments, the individual takes an extreme action that is either dangerous or outside social norms.

These **moments of madness** are to an ADHDer an appropriate response to quieten the turmoil in their heads. It's an external outlet of frustration. They don't normally result in malicious acts and are usually self-directed. Shaparak Khorsandi describes painting purple hearts on the walls of her house during a lockdown.[7] Consider them like a boiling kettle letting off steam. Stuck inside at home during the long summer holidays of

5 *Aftersun* (2022) written and directed by Charlotte Wells.
6 *The Worst Person in the World* (2021) co-written by Eskil Vogt and Joachim Trier, directed by Joachim Trier.
7 *Scatter Brain* (Shaparak Khorsandi, Vermilion, 2023).

my childhood, I'd find all sorts of (ridiculous) ways to try to fill the dopamine deficit: making complicated meals, cycling long distances, arguing with my sister, or creating expansive adventures in nearby playing fields.

While an ADHDer might sometimes take risky one-off measures to relieve boredom, they're always on the lookout for dopamine.

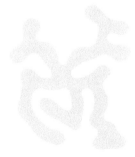

BEHAVIOURS

Dopamine Hunting

An ADHDer is on the constant lookout for ways to generate dopamine, whether they're aware of it or not. A friend who'd decided to stop taking his ADHD medication, said that as soon as one thing had sated him, he was always on the hunt for something else. It was relentless and quite difficult to listen to.

The ADHDer will keep going in the pursuit of things that gives them dopamine. Often, it's something 'interesting' e.g. a new hobby. My current passion is making electronic music and even thinking about it, makes me feel elevated. For many ADHDers, their dopamine generator is their profession.

This is a great way of managing ADHD as it's a healthy way of getting dopamine. The only risk is what to do when it no longer works. What does a musician do when no one buys their records anymore? Or a person's role changes to something less interesting? Or a sportsman can no longer perform when they were at their peak? In these situations, the ADHDer can become frustrated and even depressed. In their attempts to turn things around, they have two routes they can follow.

Since dopamine can be generated through several types of behaviour, it means there's both 'good' and 'bad' ways to get it. Hobbies are good and many an ADHDer will have multiple hobbies in their lifetime. Often, once they're good at them, or reached a plateau, they'll lose interest and move onto the next one. It's not uncommon to see the debris of hobbies scattered about an ADHDer's home. Some of these **neeks** were never even used. A specific example is **gear acquisition syndrome** (GAS) which occurs when an ADHDer buys gadgets or collectables, often music related, that never get played, used, or unboxed.

An innocuous method of acquiring dopamine is through **stimming** (derived from self-stimulation). This includes a range of activities, such as small movements (fidgeting or fiddling), scratching, foot tapping, doodling, checking phone, mumbling, or walking about. You can also buy small devices that facilitate stimming e.g. fidget cubes

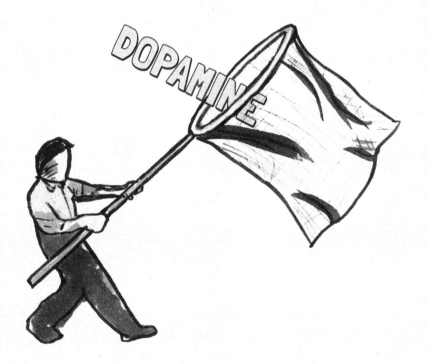

or spinners. While harmless, stimming can irritate other people and it can appear that the ADHDer is not paying attention. In fact, the opposite is true, the stimming's *helping* them concentrate.

While there are plenty of healthy ways to get dopamine e.g. sport, hobbies, even these can be taken to extremes e.g. ultra-marathons, base jumping. There are others that seem innocuous e.g. caffeine or sugar, but these too can get out of control (Bob Mortimer said he has always had a sweet tooth and would regularly have 16 sugars in his tea and coffee when he was younger). Bizarrely, caffeine makes me sleepy. As a teenager, I used to take multiple spoons of sugar in my tea. I still have a weakness for sweet and sour dishes.

One particular trait of the ADHDer is being socially outrageous. This can take several forms, the simplest may be either taking no interest in their appearance – "who can be bothered" – to dyeing their hair unusual colours or dressing extravagantly. Pink and purple seem popular. Another trait is to *say* something outrageous (**broken filter**), often when the conversation feels like its lagging. Or to avoid or skew social norms such as "How are you?" When the musician Bob Geldof met the producer Trevor Horn for the first time, Geldof immediately told Horn how he preferred the Bruce Woolley version of *Video Killed the Radio Star* to Horn's own version.[8]

Things become more serious when an ADHDer turns to alcohol, nicotine, cannabis, gambling,[9] amphetamines, opioids, and barbiturates for their dopamine fix. Of course, these chemicals have their own specific effects and can cause harm to those without ADHD. But for the ADHDer, the combined hit is extremely seductive. It can become an addiction that can lead to health complications and occasionally tragic outcomes.

As previously mentioned, GAS is a specific type of dopamine hunting and a great example of the next topic – the ADHDer's attraction to intricate squares.

---

8 *Adventures in Modern Recording: From ABC to ZTT* (Trevor Horn, Nine Eight Books, 2022).

9 https://www.england.nhs.uk/2023/07/nhs-doubles-gambling-clinics-as-referrals-soar

BEHAVIOURS

Boxes with Complexity

ADHDers seem drawn to 'boxes with complexity.' These boxes are any square or rectangular object or surface, that contains a complex or elaborate activity. The simplest example might be a board game, like snakes and ladders. Or a mobile phone game like Candy Crush or Two Dots. My father loved the word-based board game, Scrabble, and was national champion.[10]

My preference was chess. There are over three trillion ways just to play the first four moves. I got pretty good at it too, playing for Middlesex, but became bored when games took longer, and I realised that a large amount of studying was needed. This took away much of the creative element and it became more like a memory game (much like top-

---

10 He published a book on it, called *Play Better Scrabble* (Michael Goldman, Magnetical, 2019).

level Scrabble requires knowing every seven-letter word) and therefore less fun.

There are three-dimensional boxes with complexity e.g. synthesisers. With their buttons and flashing lights, they're often a magnet to anyone with ADHD. Within them lies a world of possibilities to be creative. Éliane Radigue is a pioneer of electronic music, and well-known for working with a synthesiser called the ARP 2500. This is a large analog unit made of one to two dozen interconnectable modules. Radigue talks about it like it's alive and how she discards clichéd sounds until she finds one she likes. Her face beams with happiness: "An interesting tiny little thing!"[11]

A tennis court or snooker table are good examples. A constrained playing surface with a multitude of opportunities to be creative without too much interference. And it's exercise too. Ronnie O'Sullivan is the best snooker player there's ever been. He can play with both hands. When interviewed, he's self-effacing and focuses on moments in the match rather than his achievement. He recently suggested that other (younger) players seemed to be slow of thought and often falls out with the referees and other

11 *A Portrait of Éliane Radigue* (2009) by the Austrian IMA (Institute for Media Archeology).

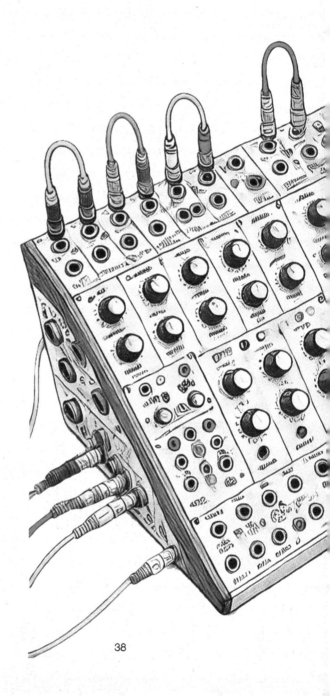

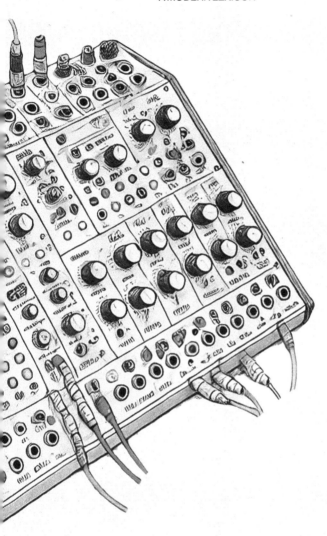

officials. A previous world champion, Steve Davis, is now fascinated by modular synthesisers. Perhaps the two of them have something in common other than snooker?

One of the most creative, talented, and controversial tennis players is Nick Kyrgios. He's well known for using the occasional underarm serve as well as his outbursts on court, often against authority. And he's complex off it too, being pleasant one minute then provocative the next. This is typical (if an extreme externalisation) of the ADHDer's brain, which can switch sides in an instance, even when they're radically opposed.

Let's go deeper in the ADHDer's ability to see both sides as well as rebel against authority.

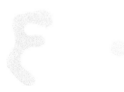

BEHAVIOURS

Duality and Opposition

An ADHDer has a unique approach to logical reasoning. While on the one hand they're great at seeing both sides of an argument, they can be drawn to the more interesting viewpoint, even if it has less merit. Aristotle believed that a well-structured argument consisted of a hypothesis, antithesis, and a synthesis. You begin by stating the hypothesis e.g., "An asteroid may one day hit the earth", an opposing statement e.g., "An asteroid will never hit the earth," and then a concluding statement considering both sides of the argument e.g., "We should prepare for an asteroid hitting the earth, even it if it doesn't, as not doing so would be catastrophic in the event that one does."

The downside of an ADHDer's ability to give equal importance to both sides of an argument is they'll struggle to pick one, which is made worse when a compromise (synthesis) doesn't exist. Trying to choose between two similar colours to paint a wall can be extremely challenging. In more complex situations, data and evidence, or advice from a friend, can help to reach a decision. But it's possible that the ADHDer will become overwhelmed and make no decision.

In some situations, an ADHDer will be drawn to the extreme position as this offers the most excitement. *The blade of a knife is the sharpest part.* I'll often find myself suggesting the most outlandish of solutions to solve a simple problem. Things can go awry when the ADHDer is drawn to extreme positions or outlandish theories such as religious fundamentalism or conspiracy theories. From Pizzagate[12] to the QAnon,[13] the US seems to have more than its fair share of conspiracy theories. And they're often associated with a mistrust of state institutions e.g. government, media.

When these beliefs are minor or not acted upon, they can be seen as a bit of fun. Whether it's believing in UFOs, faked moon landings, or lizards in power, we can all have

---

12 Pizzagate is a conspiracy theory that went viral in 2016 falsely claiming that the New York City Police Department had discovered a paedophilia ring linked to members of the Democratic Party.
13 QAnon is a conspiracy theory and political movement that originated in 2017 which believed that a cabal of Satanic cannibalistic child molesters was operating a global child sex trafficking ring that conspired against Donald Trump.

a laugh in a "What if?" kind of way. But for those who find their work diminished or their honour questioned, it can be upsetting. Buzz Aldrin punched someone who told him he never stepped onto the moon.[14] And if believed by enough people (with or without ADHD), could result in radical behaviour e.g. the US January 6th riots?[15]

So why might this trait exist? It doesn't appear to be helpful when it could result in such dramatic outcomes. Might this be the adult equivalent of **oppositional defiant disorder** – antagonistic behaviour of a child to authority? If beneficial traits persist (or increase) in line with evolutionary theory, why might this one still exist? Could it be, that occasionally, the ADHDer is correct? That injustice left unnoticed will continue e.g. the British Post Office scandal.[16] When combined with **justice sensitivity**,[17] this could manifest itself as moral outrage.

---

14 https://www.history.com/this-day-in-history/buzz-aldrin-punches-moon-landing-conspiracy-theorist-bart-sibrel

15 On 6 January 2021, a mob of Donald Trump's supporters attacked the Capitol Building in the US.

16 The Post Office pursued thousands of innocent sub-postmasters for shortfalls in their accounts, which had been caused by faults in their Fujitsu Horizon software.

17 Bondü R, Esser G. (2015) *Justice and rejection sensitivity in children and adolescents with ADHD symptoms.* Eur Child Adolesc Psychiatry. 2015 Feb; 24(2):185-98.

On 3rd October 1992, Sinéad O'Connor was scheduled to sing on *Saturday Night Live*. Instead, she tore up a photograph of Pope John Paul II in protest at the Catholic Church's denial of child sexual abuse.[18]

Nan Goldin is a successful photographer who had intimate knowledge of the US and Canada's opioid epidemic. Her campaign, documented in the film, *All the Beauty and the Bloodshed*[19] recorded how Goldin and her collaborators forced the world's leading museums and galleries to drop financial ties with the Sackler family, whose family business, Purdue Pharma developed the prescription painkiller OxyContin.

Goldin appeared to have found her **tribe**, likeminded individuals to socialise with and campaign together. But how did she find them?

---

18 https://tvline.com/news/sinead-oconnor-snl-pope-ripping-photo-video-death-1235019279/

19 *All the Beauty and the Bloodshed* (2022) directed by Laura Poitras.

BEHAVIOURS

Weirdar

There's a common term used by the gay community, **gaydar**, to describe the unscientific ability to identify a gay person. There's no formula or rulebook on how to do it. Some people just seem able to. In a similar way, I propose **weirdar**. There's something about ADHDers that we can see in others. This might be simply because of their pink hair or their tapping foot. But often it's not as *obvious* as that. If the ADHDers begin a conversation, it flows effortlessly and feels comforting.

I've spent time in LGBTQ+ circles and have observed the ease with which they socialise. There's an unwritten understanding that comes from shared experiences and similar viewpoints. It's much the same with ADHDers. Put them in a group and they feel naturally at ease. They'll talk fast and jump from topic to topic (**vibing**). While they'll normally adapt to social norms the rest of the time, being

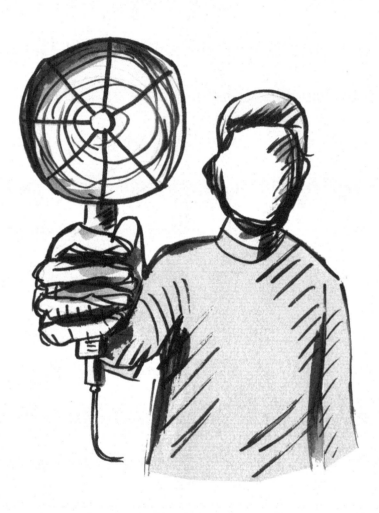

able to go full ADHD feels like finding an empty swimming pool. While I suggest weirdar as a term to use, I do so with a note of caution. I believe it's a term best kept within the ND community. I don't believe it's appropriate for NTs to be referring to ADHDers as weird.

Some ADHDers won't like the suggestion that they're weird. But I'd contest that the definitions of weird (unnatural, strange character or behaviour, fantastic, peculiar) are the descriptions that NT people use to describe ADHDers. Let's embrace it. And while inclusivity is to be encouraged, diversity must also be acknowledged. Some ADHDers might describe NTs as dull, boring, lame, and uninteresting. It's okay to be different.

One trait common to ADHDers is lateness. While never intended to cause offence, it's a behaviour that many ADHDers can't help but display.

BEHAVIOURS

"Oh Dear! Oh Dear! I Shall Be Too Late!"[20]

People with ADHD are often late. Not usually very late, but enough to annoy those waiting. This lateness is not malicious and it's normally accompanied by a heartfelt apology. The ADHDer will often feel guilt or shame about it. There are situations where we can be on time – often where the penalty of being late is to miss something (interesting), where they're the organiser, or representing someone or something else e.g. employer. On these occasions they're often extra early.

Lateness can be attributable to the difficulty of getting up early or negotiating a complex travel route. My mother was summoned to school to explain while I was always

---

20 Words spoken by the White Rabbit in *Alice's Adventures in Wonderland* (Lewis Carroll, Collins Classics, 2010).

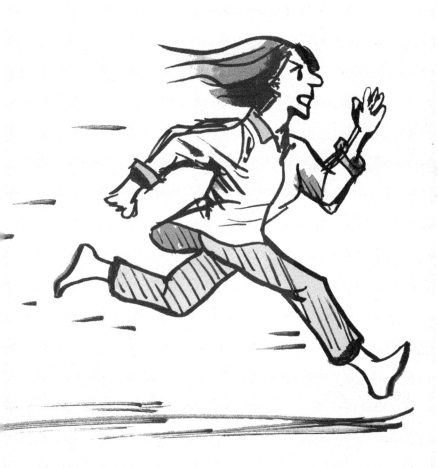

late. A school I attended as an adult had a specific answer to late arrivals – ban late arrivals from entering the class (for the first hour if it was a long class). I was told it did the trick.

Other than struggling with mornings, lateness may be in part due to the ADHDer's difficulty with time. This often manifests itself in poor judgement of how long something really takes e.g., "It'll only take ten minutes to get there, so we'll leave ten minutes before it starts?" But the ADHDer doesn't consider all the elements around the actual journey time e.g. finding a parking space. This can also apply to judging how long it'll take to complete a project e.g. an essay. And sometimes we lose complete track of what time it is (**time blindness**).

ADHDers work best with a deadline, even if they might leave the activity to the last minute. Homework's often completed the night before its due. Unless I have a slight feeling of *panic*, it's hard to gather the impetus to start something. And if the activity isn't of interest, it's even harder. Sure, it might inconvenience or annoy someone, but that often feels like a sensible trade. Missing the trailers to a film or the opening act of a play isn't that important, is it? While the ADHDer might be entertaining company, they're unreliability might mean they're not invited in the future.

When an ADHDer's about to leave home, getting ready can feel as difficult as climbing a mountain in high heels. There are *so* many distractions: the washing up, the hoovering, watering the plants. These could all be quickly completed before setting off, couldn't they? Then there's the admin required to go out: putting on shoes, picking a coat, finding their wallet, phone and keys. Invariably they'll also want to pack too much: a bottle of water in case they're thirsty (that they'll forget to drink) or something to read (which they'll never look at). And sometimes they'll be hooked into a dopamine source e.g. TV, a game, that will make it even harder to start the process.

Once we're out of the house, it's a great relief and gives them no small sense of achievement. And now that we're out, an ADHDer is going to make the most of it.

BEHAVIOURS

One More Thing

Now we're out, we don't want to come back. Once we're out, we're presented with numerous sources of interest (e.g. dopamine): people, architecture, traffic, noise, weather. It's a playground. ADHDers are full of energy, observant, and always thinking about what fun thing they can do next.

The ADHDer might plan a day that's a mixture of fun activities and tasks (although they'll often wing it). Having some interesting ones as a reward can help to get errands completed: "I'll take the rubbish to the dump, then go for a pub lunch." But equally we might just go out to do one thing and find the thought of going straight home dull. Every crossroads offers an alternative direction.

When an ADHDer is out, they're great organisers and no one's better at keeping the party going. They can move from one venue to another, one bar to the next, without hesitation (or thought of the cost). The ADHDer keeps the dopamine flowing. After an hour or two in one cafe or bar, itchy feet will start to drag them up and away to somewhere else. As the day or night progresses, we might find ourselves so overstimulated that we head home. Alternatively, we might seek more thrills and take riskier choices.

An ADHDer seems to have a lower threshold for danger or at least, it seems to reduce when the demand for one more dopamine hit becomes too powerful to resist. Even when I've got lost in foreign cities late at night, one thing that hasn't deserted me is being alert to danger.

BEHAVIOURS

Hey! Look, a Squirrel

Some believe that ADHD exists because it benefits society. When we lived in small communities, we were at risk of attack from other tribes, the odd hungry carnivore would hunt for meat. In these more dangerous times, an ADHDer was the ideal candidate to take on the dual role of hunter and protector.[21]

An ADHDer is willing to take risks, they're awake late at night, and they spot danger quickly. While the chapter title is tongue-in-cheek, I did once spot two baby squirrels chasing each other on the side of a tree out of the corner of my eye. I often spot odd things that no one else has. Is this a consequence of a faster brain? Better peripheral vision? Or because ADHDers are attuned to danger?

---

21 *ADHD: A Hunter in a Farmer's World* (Thom Hartmann, Healing Arts Press, 2019).

While an ADHDer might be ideally suited as a night watch, their quick reactions make them excellent hunters. NTs make excellent farmers where methodical, forward thinking is required. But when meat was needed for the village, who better to go into the dark forest than an ADHDer. They'd have picked up spear throwing in no time and would be quick to spot a boar darting through a bush.

In our safer modern world,[22] there's less need for an ADHDer to be patrolling the neighbourhood or hunting. So what good are these abilities now? Unfortunately, the world is still full of crises whether it be wars, famine, or traffic accidents. When emergencies occur, the ADHDer can swing into action. They're keen and can use their fast thinking and observational skills to help.

ADHDers also envisage the unthinkable, often sensing danger or predicting disasters. Maybe it's a pattern recognition ability or just our anxious natures? Whatever it is, the ADHDer seems to be always alert, on the move even if they're often bumping into things. Indeed, their busy bee nature is best exemplified by how they deal with tasks.

---

22 In 1900, the average life expectancy was 32 years, a hundred years later it was 72. https://ourworldindata.org/life-expectancy

BEHAVIOURS

Zigzagging

The term zigzagging describes the way an ADHDer will complete tasks in disjointed small steps. Usually, these tasks are boring or repetitive. To combat this, the ADHDer will start one, then switch to another, then may come back to the first one, but might also start a third. They may or may not finish any of the tasks they started.

I hate unloading the dishwasher. When I do it, I'll usually take everything out and lay it on the worktop. Then I do something else. Twenty minutes later, I'll put most of it away, sweeping the cutlery haphazardly into the drawer. Later or even the next day, I'll segregate the forks, knives, and spoons into their allocated trays. The remaining saucepan may sit there for another day or two.

Zigzagging is a relatively innocuous behaviour, particularly if you live or work alone. For those who don't, it might be

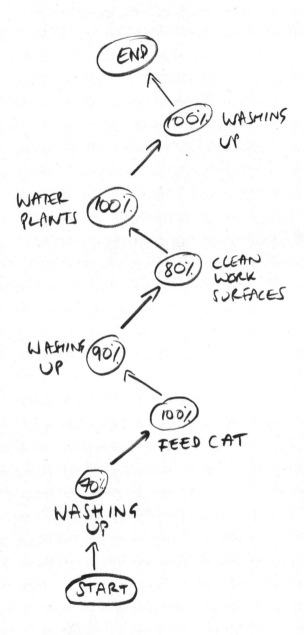

annoying to others. It should've become apparent how many of these ADHD behaviours can annoy NTs. But there are many NT-ND relationships that function well. Perhaps the ADHDer loads and unloads the dishwasher, and the NT puts stuff away? Zigzagging does get these tasks done, eventually, even if it might look odd.

While zigzagging is a great technique for ADHDers to complete chores like housework, it doesn't work for something more complicated. That requires deep thought and concentration. For that an ADHDer needs something else.

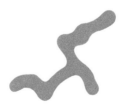

BEHAVIOURS

Hyperfocus

Hyperfocus describes an ADHDer's ability to concentrate intensely on a topic, often for an extended period. This will be something that interests them. They may do this simply as it's pleasurable to be immersed in a hobby. If they've found a new 'love', it can be extremely intoxicating. When I was a child, I loved chess and would happily spend hours at a tournament. My feet used to get so cold, I'd wear thick woollen socks. I'd be so absorbed the rest of the world would disappear.

Hyperfocus is an extremely helpful tool for an ADHDer's poor ability to manage deadlines. They can meet them, but usually at the last minute. Hyperfocus allows them to sprint to the finish line, having been several laps behind.[23]

---

23 In *Adventures in Modern Recording: From ABC to ZTT*, Horn describes how to meet a deadline, he went for "thirty-six hours relying purely on coffee".

But in doing so they'll ignore everything or everyone around them as well as forgetting to eat or drink.

Hyperfocus is often referred to as a *superpower* (as are some other ADHD traits), but it rarely feels like one. Maybe because it feels like they've no choice but to use it. It can sometimes feel like a treadmill going too fast, with a looming comedown to follow when the task is complete. Like committing to a heavy night's drinking, we know there'll be an almighty hangover. However, when there's no deadline and hyperfocus kicks in, it feels like catching the perfect wave.

ADHD brains are structurally and functionally different to NT ones.[24] Often it feels like I've two Central Processing Units (CPUs) rather than one or two faders on an audio mixer. Most of the time, only one is working while the other is hibernating or looking for more interesting things than what's currently the focus of attention. Sometimes, they'll work together, performing like a single, heavily overclocked single CPU. They'll run faster than an ordinary CPU but likely to overheat and burn out.

24 Firouzabadi FD, Ramezanpour S, Firouzabadi MD, Yousem IJ, Puts NAJ, Yousem DM. (2022) *Neuroimaging in Attention-Deficit/Hyperactivity Disorder: Recent Advances*. AJR Am J Roentgenol. 2022 Feb; 218(2):321-332.

In this split-brain model, each side feels like its fighting for attention. If I'm lucky, the dominant one is focussed on what's important e.g. listening to instructions. But if it loses interest, the other half takes dominance, with flights of fancy: "What's going on outside? I wonder if anyone's texted me?" The two halves can sometimes find a happy medium. For example, at a concert I'll be listening to the music but at the same time dreaming up t-shirt slogans.

An ADHDer's life becomes difficult when the second stream takes over too often. The ADHDer becomes the classic *dreamer staring out of the window*. At this point, performance of any task takes a nosedive. This can result in poor school results, missing vital instructions about a work task, or tripping over.

When an ADHDer starts a task or an activity they're interested in, they fully intend to finish it. Hyperfocus can help but there's a looming problem – the 'last mile'.

BEHAVIOURS

The Last Mile

ADHDers can struggle to complete tasks. I think for the most part this is related to boredom and is prevalent when no one else is waiting on the output. If an ADHDer needs to complete a task that's uninteresting, they'll have

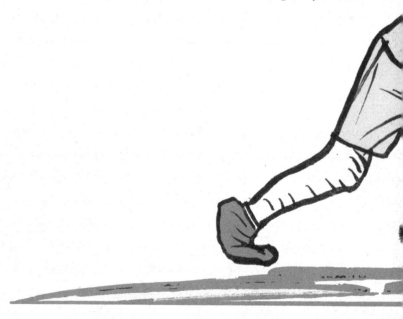

enough *oomph* to get most of it done but often be unable to finish it. An ADHDer might start vacuuming but give up after a couple of rooms. On a recent holiday, my inability to cover all my exposed skin with insect repellent resulted in multiple bites.

The last element of a task feels like a step too far. I'm pretty good at deciding I now no longer need something

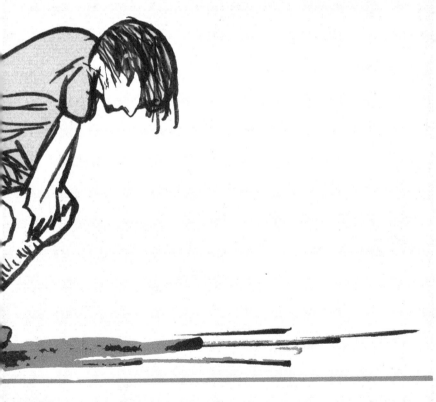

but the process of selling it feels like too much admin, so it usually goes to charity. While many activities left uncompleted are not vital, some can be e.g. a tax return, MOT renewal.

Leaving something unfinished manifests itself in other ways. ADHDers often leave a bit of food or drink uneaten. It takes a significant effort for me to drink something right down to the bottom. It doesn't help that because I'd forgotten about it, it's now cold. Does this matter? Not to me, but it can annoy others. In a restaurant or cafe, they'll probably say nothing but as a child told to clean their plate, it's painful.

When an ADHDer doesn't finish something, often it goes unnoticed. The ADHDer will likely still feel some internal shame or disappointment: "It's happened again". But when it's noticed, it can result in criticism, poor marks or damaged relationships. Another element that impacts an ADHDer's ability to complete a task, is that they didn't fully listen to or understand what the necessary requirements were to complete it in the first place.

BEHAVIOURS

Memory

ADHDers have impaired memory function.[25] Specifically, the way an ADHDer stores memories is worse for verbal events compared to visual ones. I only remember what I find interesting, particularly if there was a strong visual element. My recollection will be quite different to others at the same event. If I had a conversation with someone, I may remember none of it, whereas they'll usually remember something.

Many times, the memory will be the same for us all (NT and ND), such as recalling the moment the team we support scored a goal or when a child is born. But many times, it isn't. Does this matter? It depends. ADHDers are

25 Skodzik T, Holling H, Pedersen A. (2017) *Long-Term Memory Performance in Adult ADHD*. Journal of Attention Disorders. 2017 Feb; 21(4), 267-283.

great raconteurs, recalling funny or amazing incidents, one after the other. But ask an ADHDer to accurately recount a dull but important list of instructions – *little to no chance*. Any activity that becomes uninteresting, dissipates from memory. I might start with a hot cup of fragrant tea, but it's soon forgotten about it and becomes a cold, brown soup.

An ADHDer's desire for interesting moments can affect their behaviour. ADHDers will be attracted to social events and add sparkle to them, sometimes literally, by dressing extravagantly. When playing cricket, I'd be keener to bowl tricky deliveries than bread and butter ones. If any of them came off, they'd stick in the memory far more than if we won or lost. After a snooker tournament in 2023, Ronnie O'Sullivan said about trophies, "I always give them away." The creative moment was the most rewarding element. The artist Dorothea Rockburne[26] said, "I don't really like goals, they seem like the end of something. I'm much more interested in process."

The negative consequence of focussing on the journey rather than the outcome is that you might not get to

---

26 *Bauhaus Spirit: 100 Years of Bauhaus* (2018) by Signature Entertainment.

the end. It also doesn't align with societal measures of success. Much of life is about winning or completing tasks, not about the *way* they were completed. Bosses often overlook shortcuts or rules broken if an urgent task gets finished on time. ADHDers often meander and don't prioritise the task in hand. When Thomas Dolby, a musician and entrepreneur, talked about his time as a CEO, he said that his *flights of fancy* might've been to the detriment of his business.[27]

Despite an ADHDer's poor memory along with all the other challenges in completing a task well and on time, they'll still seek perfection.

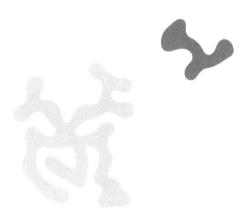

27 In his book, *The Speed of Sound: Breaking the Barriers Between Music and Technology: a Memoir* (Thomas Dolby, Flatiron Books, 2016).

BEHAVIOURS

Perfection

While there may be no such thing as perfection, that doesn't mean an ADHDer won't strive for it. When an ADHDer cares about something e.g. a new interest, they can score high marks or succeed in the workplace. An ADHDer may complete the work at the last minute, but it'll get done. An ADHDer will often strive for perfection, forgetting that they're not well designed for it. For example, when writing a report, they'll often make silly spelling or grammatical mistakes or miss an instruction.

An ADHDer's desire for perfection can compound their difficulty in meeting a deadline. Often, the activities that they seek to perfect are the ones that they have the most interest in. Radigue, the French musician, said that if she made a mistake in the 75th minute of an 80-minute piece, she'd have to start again. I've seen Damon Michael Gough, the musician known as Badly Drawn Boy, restart several songs in a single concert.

This desire for perfection can also make decision making difficult, particularly between two similar choices or where there's little information or it's complex. For me, choosing paint colours for my home took many months of agonising. An ADHDer's life can be full of frustrations because of their brains being wired differently and the world being set up for NTs. There are some things we really don't like.

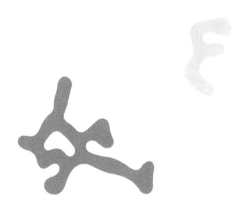

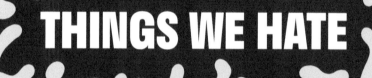
THINGS WE HATE

THINGS WE HATE

Admin

One of the most difficult things for an ADHDer is admin (administrative tasks). It's tedious and boring. Even with self-awareness, it doesn't get any easier. It feels like rubbing sandpaper over my brain. Despite this, sometimes there's no escape from it. But the rest of the time, ADHDers don't do it, or try it and make a mess of it. They'll leave unpaid bills in **doom piles** – towers of envelopes and flyers that threaten to collapse at any moment.

The cause of this inability to do admin is called **executive dysfunction**. It covers not just admin tasks but other challenges e.g. paying attention or managing time. The consequences of not completing an admin task are missed opportunities e.g. work, funding, important information, or penalties, such as fines. Some refer to this as the **ADHD tax**. It's estimated at being about £1,600/year.[28]

28 https://monzo.com/blog/the-extra-costs-of-living-with-adhd

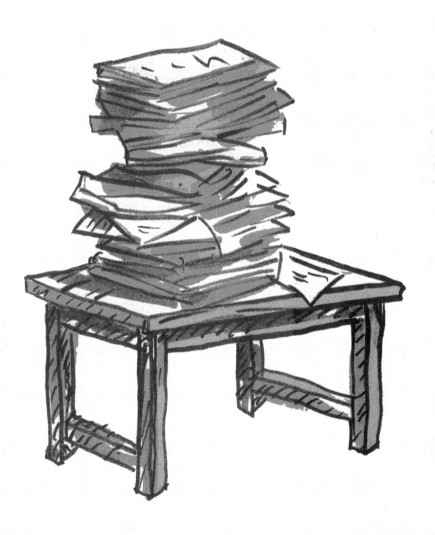

An ADHDer might forget to pay a bill, such as a parking fine, and find the penalty's doubled. Or they might buy something on impulse they don't need and will never use. The realisation that they've missed a deadline or bought something superfluous, can trigger feelings of self-loathing and guilt. This is hard to solve and something that ADHDers live with.

The challenge of admin can be mitigated against. Switching payments to direct debits and paperless billing can help. The Buddy System (see page 84) works for some either by asking or paying someone else to either complete the task or be present while the ADHDer does it themselves. For me, having someone help with my schedule is useful. For much of the time, an ADHDer can feel like they've forgotten something or are about to let someone down.

When we do manage to achieve an admin task it does feel good. If it's an application, we'll wait with bated breath for the response because one thing an ADHDer doesn't like is bad feedback.

THINGS WE HATE

Feedback

Many ADHDers struggle with feedback, especially when it's a full-on rejection. While likely to be an inherent trait, it may also be triggered by past trauma e.g. an ADHDer being told as a child they've got things wrong. **Rejection sensitive dysphoria** is a condition where someone experiences *emotional pain* because they feel like they've failed or are being rejected. Studies estimate that 35% to 70% of people with ADHD struggle with **emotional dysregulation**.[29] Emotional dysregulation manifests itself when an individual, swamped in negative feelings, resorts to self-harming behaviours.

For me, sharing my creative output (e.g. this book) puts me at the mercy of criticism. Negative feedback is hard to take

---

29 Soler-Gutiérrez AM, Pérez-González JC, Mayas J. (2023) *Evidence of emotion dysregulation as a core symptom of adult ADHD: A systematic review.* PLoS One. 2023 Jan 6; 18(1):e0280131.

rationally. An ADHDer might go into a slump, swearing never to put themselves in that situation again, be it a relationship or entering a competition. The fact that many ADHDers end up in creative fields, where competition is fierce and funding limited, can lead to depressive symptoms and low self-esteem.

For an ADHDer who's been told off for misunderstanding a task or not paying attention, that trauma is often carried with them like a wound that's failed to heal. While many will battle on, seeking validity in their personal or professional lives, the impact of the past failures can inhibit their eagerness to try and try again. But this can be overcome, both through repeated attempts but also with a greater self-awareness, the ADHDer can take the time to heal and learn ways that they can be a success.

One is the Poison King method (mithridatism).[30] It's been said that some kings, with fear for their lives through poisoning, would take a small amount every day to make them immune to attack. We can do this in a similar way by repeated attempts at whatever we wish to thrive at.

---

30 *The Poison King: The Life and Legend of Mithradates, Rome's Deadliest Enemy* (Adrienne Mayor, Princeton University Press, 2009).

For example, I've a spreadsheet with about three hundred competitions or funding submissions. Most resulted in rejections. But with so many entries completed, each new rejection hurts a bit less.

While I might never meet the person receiving my application, there's one type of person it's hard to avoid.

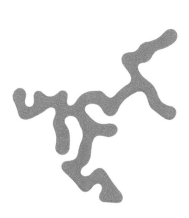

THINGS WE HATE

Bosses

ADHDers rarely like bosses. You'll normally either find an ADHDer either working for themselves[31] or in a role with plenty of autonomy. But it doesn't stop an ADHDer running a business with employees. It will be hard – businesses usually require a lot of administration for a start – but there are well known examples e.g. Sir Richard Branson (business magnate), Ingvar Kamprad (IKEA founder), and David Neeleman (aviation entrepreneur).

Many ADHDers have likely unwittingly found ways to help themselves, such as having an (NT) business partner. Or they may be more conscious of their strengths and weaknesses and employ people to help them. I've seen an inventor with

---

31 Verheul I, Rietdijk W, Block J, Franken I, Larsson H, Thurik R. (2016) *The association between attention deficit/hyperactivity (ADHD) symptoms and self-employment.* Eur J Epidemiol. 2016 Aug; 31(8):793-801.

a whole team of freelancers and subcontractors making their vision a reality.

For many ADHDers, freelancing is their best option. The ADHDer usually has the freedom to choose their work schedules, to complete tasks in their own way, but still has that steadying influence of an outside force providing direction, positive feedback and most importantly, deadlines. When an ADHDer is employed, it can be a challenge if their boss and colleagues are NT. With traditional workplaces set up for them, an ADHDer must fit in with their behaviour, often masking to get by. And when they don't, they can be side-lined or even admonished.

Working as a freelancer gives the ADHDer plenty of freedom to structure the day in a way that suits them. This can include starting later.

Getting Up Early

Getting up early can be tough for an ADHDer. It's like being a teenager all over again, with a parent shouting through the bedroom door, telling them to get up. An ADHDer will go to sleep later[32] and have poorer sleep.[33] An ADHDer is at their most alert in the afternoon or evening and often called a 'night' person. It might contribute to why it seems that so many musicians and comedians are recently being diagnosed with ADHD.

In today's more flexible work environment, being someone who starts work late is less of a problem. But

---

32 Kooij JJ, Bijlenga D. (2013) *The circadian rhythm in adult attention-deficit/ hyperactivity disorder: current state of affairs.* Expert Rev Neurother. 2013 Oct; 13(10):1107-16.

33 Van Veen MM, Kooij JJ, Boonstra AM, Gordijn MC, Van Someren EJ. (2010) *Delayed circadian rhythm in adults with attention-deficit/hyperactivity disorder and chronic sleep-onset insomnia.* Biol Psychiatry. 2010 Feb; 67(11):1091-6.

for me as a child, arriving at school on time was a real challenge. Even as an adult, getting into the workplace before ten o'clock is tough. And if am, I tend to be grumpy and non-communicative for at least an hour. Help is available such as getting educated on good sleep routines, by taking melatonin or using bright light therapy in the morning.

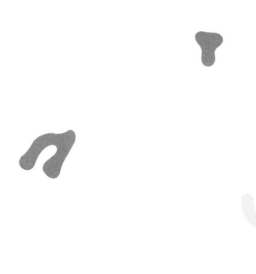

COPING METHODS

COPING METHODS

The Buddy System

A buddy is a person, usually an NT, who acts as anchor to provide stability. This is somewhat different from a scuba diving 'buddy', where the principal purpose is to provide safety. An ADHD buddy is like a flagpole to the flag or the string to a kite, allowing an ADHDer to move and think freely but without going too far. The buddy provides stability in an ADHDer's life.

A buddy can bring an ADHDer back to reality. When an ADHDer organising a networking event for a group of accountants might feel it would benefit from a troop of fire jugglers, their buddy will persuade them that it's not really suitable. Every Bob Geldof needs a Midge Ure just like Homer needs Marge.

A buddy may also provide a more mundane purpose. While they provide a secure point for the ADHDer to let loose,

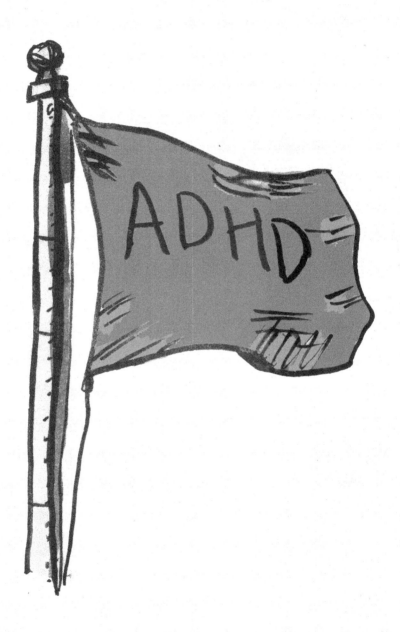

the buddy relationship has other benefits. A buddy could perform administrative tasks for the ADHDer. This could be filling in a form, researching a council website, or posting a parcel. A buddy can also be helpful in a less direct way – as a steadying presence (**body doubling**) while the ADHDer attempts the task themselves. The buddy may simply have to sit nearby to help get the task done.

When an ADHDer doesn't have a buddy or hasn't found a lifestyle that works, they'll often consider a dramatic solution.

COPING METHODS

The Oasis

When you know people with ADHD, you may get used to their behaviour. They're exciting: always busy, with many interests and always going out. But sometimes their lives can look like a chaotic mess. Occasionally, an ADHDer might find a peaceful nirvana – free of distractions and temptations. This oasis can take several forms: the cottage in the country, a caravan in Cornwall, or simply stripping back their life to the essentials: working, eating, and sleeping.

The oasis for an ADHDer may sound like a fanciful pursuit but it does work for some. Free of the complexity of modern life, it can be a respite. ADHDers can wax lyrical about leaving it all to live on an island. But can this work? I think so if they can find ways to get their dopamine fix e.g. having family nearby, lots of pets, or nature on their doorstep.

But for many, it's a fantasy that fails to deliver what they need. The hope that simplicity might lead to a stillness in their heads proves unfounded. When they've got used to their new environment, it's no longer new. And having fewer choices of things to do becomes restrictive. A recently decorated home no longer has the potential for creative enhancement.

I spent a month in Berlin to attend a music course. Many of my fellow students had ADHD. One thing that struck me was their extreme reactions to it compared to those who were NT. Several said it was the best place they'd ever been – the school and the city – with a few saying they were going to move to Berlin permanently. But by the end of the month, the gloss had worn off for several of them.

Whether an ADHDer might find somewhere free of distractions, or a 24-hour playground, living on a real or virtual island isn't practical for most people. For those living a more conventional existence, they may look for solutions closer to home.

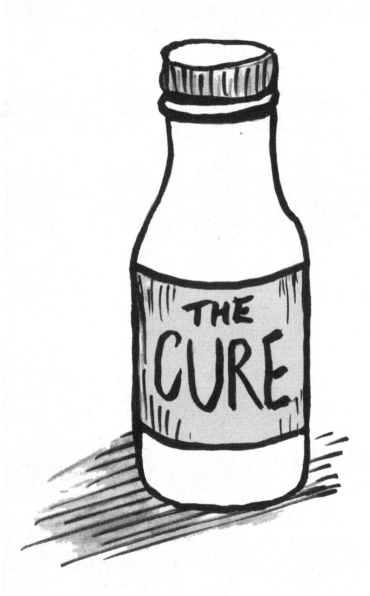

COPING METHODS

Secret Sauce

The disabling impacts of ADHD can be so challenging that an ADHDer may look for a quick fix. Their frustration with the ease with which others (NTs usually) navigate the world can make them grab for something out of desperation. Most of these rash attempts are unsustainable. However, while some can provide a long-term solution, such as the right medication, they don't work for every ADHDer.

My ADHD is mild, and medication would likely have a net negative effect on my health. Others I know do benefit from ADHD drugs. There are non-prescription options, but most are typical of a healthy lifestyle e.g. nutritious food, no or low amounts of alcohol, meditation, regular exercise and good sleep hygiene. Some ADHDers go further, seeking the help of lifestyle gurus, embracing positive-thinking, or weekend retreats spent fire walking.

While these can give anyone a boost of confidence, the benefits to the ADHDer seem short-lived.

In the next section, I'll summarise some things that could be helpful.

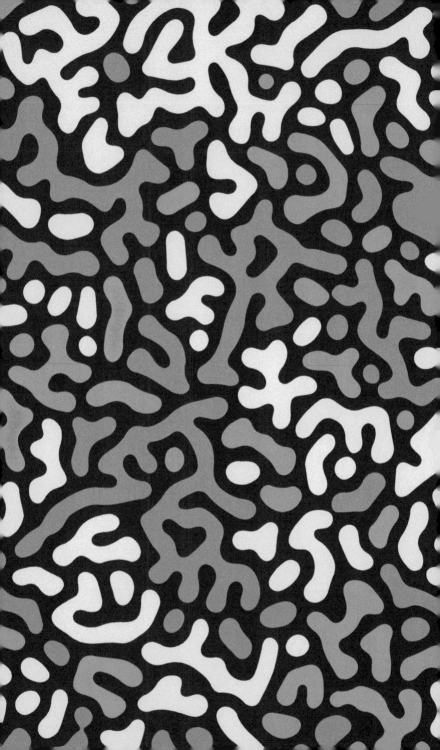

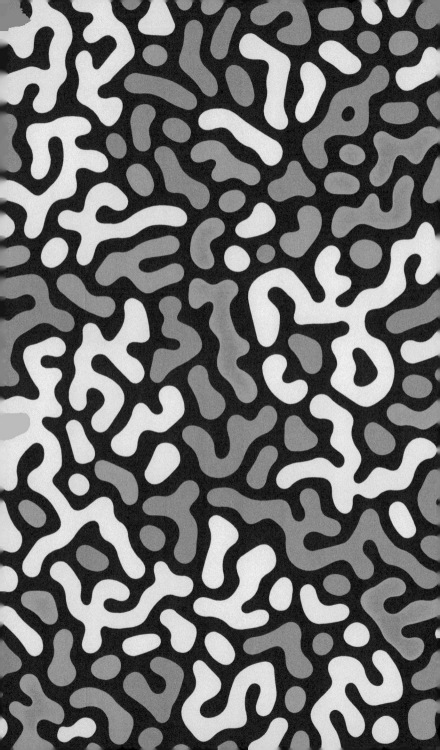

TIPS AND TRICKS

Here are a few tips and tricks I've picked up or seen others use to good effect:

FOOD

- Eat healthily.
- Supplements focussed on mental and gut health e.g. fish oil, CBD, probiotics.
- Make your own kefir.

SLEEP

- Reduce screen time before bed.
- Go to bed when tired and relaxed.
- Get up when you've had enough.
- Try melatonin or bright light therapy.

EXERCISE

- Do something every day.
- Vary activity to avoid boredom.

WORK

- Find a role with autonomy.
- Work as a freelancer.

ROUTINE

- Find a routine that works (which still has variety within it).
- Get some morning light.
- Work somewhere that fits the activity.
- Use music or earphones to help concentration.
- For repeating tasks, create and record the process.
- Find or create templates to make it easier to start an administrative task.
- Set milestones, deadlines, and reminders.

BUDDY UP

- Delegate tasks e.g. admin to others.
- Use friends or voice assistants.
- Body double with friends or strangers.

TIME

- Clocks. Everywhere.
- Set reminders and timers.
- Record diary invitations immediately.

TASKS

- If they feel doable, do them straight away.
- Make them interesting.
- Ask or pay someone else.

MENTAL HEALTH

- All the above.
- Talk to someone.
- Meditate or practise mindfulness.
- Breathe.

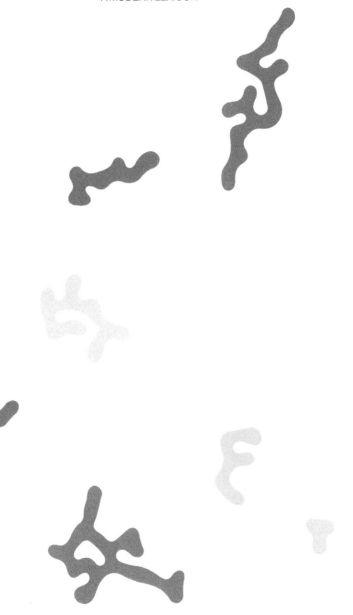

97

F.A.K.

With greater awareness of neurodiversity, schools and workplaces are increasingly making adjustments for those with ADHD to thrive. And modifications for those with any neurodivergence shouldn't negatively impact anyone else. I believe that these changes can be neatly summarised as a hierarchy of action: F.A.K.

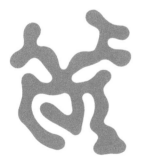

Flexibility

Provide a flexible work or study environment. This could include allowing interviewees to see the interview questions before hand. Or allow practical tests instead of written ones. Perhaps a submission could be given as a video rather than an essay.

Adjustments

Take flexibility to the next level and make those one-off exceptions, permanent adjustments. Put in place systems and measures that allow an ADHDer to work successfully. Let them work from home, start and finish later, hot desk in different locations, listen to music at their desk.

Knowledge

Understand yourself better and if you're not an ADHDer, learn about it. There are plenty of resources from books to websites e.g. adhduk.co.uk, additudemag.com. If you're a manager, try to learn from your employees with ADHD what it's like and how things could be adapted to suit them.

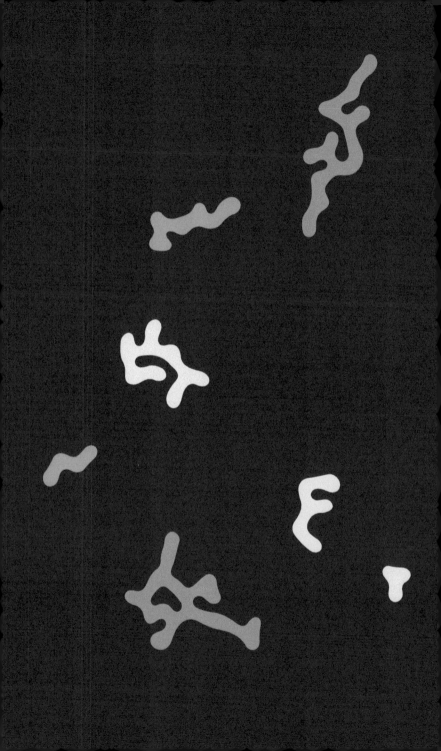

Conclusion

So, there we have it, 25 short chapters on ADHD. Hopefully, it's been an enjoyable insight if you have ADHD or not. Whether you're on your own or someone else's journey with ADHD, I wish you well.

Glossary

ADD: attention deficit disorder

ADHD tax: the financial cost of having ADHD

ADHD: attention deficit hyperactivity disorder

ADHDer: someone with ADHD

Admin: administrative tasks

ASD: autism spectrum disorder

A-Team: a group of people with ADHD*

Body doubling: working in the presence of another person

Broken filter: saying something shocking or outrageous

Doom piles: towers of unfiled paperwork, often bills

Doomscrolling: a prolonged period of scrolling downwards on an electronic device

Dopamine: 3,4-dihydroxyphenethylamine

DX: shorthand for diagnosis*

Emotional dysregulation: an inability to flexibly respond to and manage emotional states, resulting in intense and prolonged emotional reactions that deviate from social norms

Executive dysfunction: difficulties in planning, paying attention or managing time

Gaydar: the supposed ability to identify people as being gay by intuition or trivial indications

Gear acquisition syndrome: the excessive purchase of equipment, usually music related

Justice sensitivity: an increased empathy for victims of injustice

Masking: when an ND suppresses their natural behaviour and mimics an NT

Memes: funny images, often with text

Moments of madness: when an ADHDer takes a risky decision or action

Motivational salience: a cognitive process that drives us to complete a task and receive dopamine

ND: neurodivergent

Neek: an idea, invention, or activity that hasn't been executed

Neurospicy: a group of mixed neurodivergencies, often living or working together*

NHS: National Health Service

NT: neurotypical

Oppositional defiant disorder: exhibited by children, they're uncooperative, defiant and hostile toward authority figures

Pebbling: sending a meme to a friend or loved one*

Rejection sensitive dysphoria: a feeling of severe emotional pain because of a failure or feeling rejected

Ritalin: brand name for methylphenidate

Serotonin: 5-hydroxytryptamine

Stimming: small, physical movements to self-generate dopamine

Time blindness: difficulty in judging how much time has passed or how long tasks or activities will take

Touch sensitivity: needing to clean hands between activities*

Tribe: a group of individuals with a common interest

Vibing: a free-flowing conversation between NDs

Weirdar: the ability of NDs to recognise each other

*not mentioned in text

The author would like to thank all those who have helped to support the writing and publication of this book.
In particular, I'd like to thank the encouragement of the Bristol writing community and all the ADHDers I know, have met, or observed from afar.

First published 2024 by Miracle Fish

Paperback ISBN: 978-1-7384109-1-0

DALL-E was used to generate the image of the modular synthesiser prior to editing. All other images were hand drawn and shaded before being digitally coloured and edited using Pixelmator Pro.

A catalogue record for this book is available from the British Library.

Illustrations by Merlin Goldman
Designed by James Pople
Edited and proofread by Joanna Peios
Printed and bound by Ingram Spark

Country **Roads** *of*

TEXAS

Drives, Day Trips, and Weekend Excursions

Second Edition

Eleanor Morris

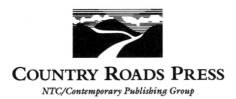

COUNTRY ROADS PRESS

NTC/Contemporary Publishing Group

Library of Congress Cataloging-in-Publication Data

Morris, Eleanor, 1944–
    Country roads of Texas : drives, day trips, and weekend excursions
/ Eleanor Morris. — 2nd ed.
      p.   cm. — (Country roads)
    Includes index.
    ISBN 1-56626-107-4
    1. Texas—Tours.   2. Automobile travel—Texas—Guidebooks.
    3. Rural roads—Texas—Guidebooks.   I. Title.   II. Series.
    F384.3.M675   1998
    917.6404'63—dc21   98-34145
                                                    CIP

Cover and interior design by Nick Panos
Cover illustration copyright © Todd L. W. Doney
Interior illustrations copyright © Barbara Kelley

Published by Country Roads Press
A division of NTC/Contemporary Publishing Group, Inc.
4255 West Touhy Avenue, Lincolnwood (Chicago), Illinois 60646-1975 U.S.A.
Copyright © 1999, 1994 by Eleanor S. Morris
Printed in the United States of America
International Standard Book Number: 1-56626-107-4

98 99 00 01 02 03 ML 18 17 16 15 14 13 12 11 10 9 8 7 6 5 4 3 2 1

To my husband, Herm

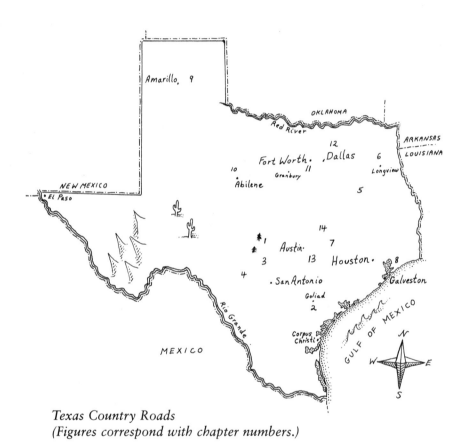

Texas Country Roads
(Figures correspond with chapter numbers.)

Contents

Introduction

I'd like to dedicate *Country Roads of Texas* to my intrepid chauffeur and companion, my husband, Herm, who (lucky me) likes to drive. He absolutely comes alive behind the wheel of a car, and although he likes to push his driving speed to the limit, he was unfailingly patient and calm in response to my shouts of "Wait!" "Stop!" "Slow down!" or "Turn around!"

Driving the small country roads of our big state of Texas turned out to be an adventure for both of us, a leisurely change from charging along superhighways in a hurry to cover large distances. It opened our eyes to what we'd been missing, to wonderful country sights that we hadn't known were there all the time.

I know it was as much fun for him as it was for me because many a weekend he'd be the one to pull out the map and say, "Well, where would you like to go next?"

He really got into the spirit of the search. How he loved sighting something he thought I'd missed. "Look at that!" he'd shout and point. (True, this usually happened as he was shooting past, but he'd turn around eagerly so we could take a look, and see if it was something our readers would want to stop and explore, too.) This happened often enough to make me really appreciate his interest in our jaunts along the back roads of Texas.

So I have high hopes that the readers of this book will be as fired up as we were with the adventure of taking to picturesque country roads. It's a relaxing and fascinating pastime, seeing what you can find while these country sights are still around to be seen. Thanks to progress, they might not be here forever.

To help clarify road designations, I've used the following abbreviations: I = Interstate, U.S. = U.S. route or highway, State = state route or highway, and FM = farm-to-market or ranch road.

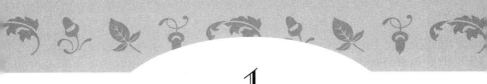

1

The Highland Lakes Trail

Getting there: This trip focuses on the chain of Highland Lakes. Take I-35 north from Austin to Round Rock (about 18 miles). Exit west on FM 1431. To return to I-35 you can take Highway 29 east or Highway 71 south to U.S. 290 east to I-35.

Highlights: Marble Falls, LBJ, Inks, and Buchanan Lakes; Marble Falls; granite quarry and Bluebonnet Cafe in Marble Falls; Inks Lake State Park and Longhorn Cavern; Fort Croghan; Burnet town square; Fall Creek Vineyards; and Llano, famous for llanite, rare rock found nowhere else in the world.

The craggy rocks of the Llano Uplift, and the pleasant blue lakes those rocks define, form one of the most interesting areas of the big state of Texas. Great land upheavals, climate variations, and the rise and fall of many prehistoric seas more than 450 billion years ago formed huge deposits of limestone, creating Longhorn Cavern and the granite that is still quarried in the area today. The countryside is especially popular in the spring, when the famous Texas wildflowers are a marvel to behold.

Then, especially on weekends, tourists are out in droves, armed with mighty cameras to record the rich palette of nature's colors: bluebonnets (state flower), red Indian paintbrush, yellow bladderwort, purple spiderwort, pink primrose, burgundy winecup, white poppies.

Driving toward Marble Falls on FM 1431, we saw breathtaking scenery both northwest and southwest as we navigated winding hills and curves, catching frequent glimpses of the Highland Lakes glinting in the sun along the way. The chain of lakes was formed by the damming of the Colorado River, and Marble Falls was named for the waterfall over the cliffs, although there is more granite than marble here.

We knew better than to look for the waterfall, though; it was covered when the lake was created. But we enjoyed seeing a picture of it in the Bluebonnet Cafe, which for more than 60 years has been a haven for both delicious and generous portions of down-home country cooking. We always try to get there around lunchtime to sample such old-time fare as pot roast, meat loaf, chicken and dumplings, thick, rich cream of cauliflower soup, and a renowned long roster of homemade pies. In addition to the more usual apple, peach, and lemon, our favorites are the peanut butter and German chocolate pies.

To Adam R. Johnson, the town's founder, the area seemed to offer a lot of potential, and as early as 1850 he began to buy up property. But along came the Civil War to interrupt his plans. He became a Confederate general but unfortunately was blinded in the war.

This did not interfere with his inner vision for the town, however, and by offering some of his land as a right-of-way for a railroad to haul the plentiful granite, he put Marble Falls on the map around 1887.

As we entered town on FM 1431, we took a slight detour south on U.S. 281 to take a look at a roadside park with a panoramic view of the lake and the town. A roadside marker there commemorates songwriter Oscar Fox: the area inspired him to write "The Hills of Home."

We backtracked on U.S. 281 to FM 1431 and turned west; we wanted to see the huge, pink mound, 866 feet high, of Granite Mountain and the quarry, the very one that in the late 1880s furnished pink granite for the Texas capitol in Austin. The quarry is not open to visitors, but huge blocks of pink granite and the cranes that lift them are visible from the road.

Other sites of historic interest we saw in Marble Falls include the Roper Hotel (now an office building), directly behind the Bluebonnet Cafe. It's on the National Register of Historic Places. Two other historic sites are not open to the public, but of course we stopped by to admire the exteriors. The Brandt Badger House is of interest because the two-story structure was built totally from the rubble left over from the shaping of the granite blocks used in building the Texas capitol. The Governor O. M. Roberts Cottage was the home of Oral M. Roberts, governor of Texas from 1879 to 1883. After he left office, he taught law at the University of Texas, retiring to this cottage in 1893.

If you're interested in old tombstones, farther along on 1431 you'll want to stop at the small Wolf Crossing Cemetery on the right, with interesting old headstones standing amid green weeds. In spring they're adorned with wildflowers.

Continuing on through Granite Shoals, a busy resort town popular with fishermen and water sports enthusiasts, we stopped to admire the fine overview of Kingsland and Lake LBJ (originally named Granite Shoals Lake) to our right, with towering limestone cliffs bordering the road. In the distance we could also see Packsaddle Mountain, site of a famous Indian battle.

To take a look at Kingsland, we continued on FM 1431. Kingsland was a popular spot for fishing even before the lakes were built, although nothing much happened until the railroad—and a general store—came in 1892. Then the railroad began to bring the fishermen around the turn of the century. The railroad even opened a hotel, the Antlers, to accommodate those it brought from Austin on fishing excursions. When the railroad quit, Kingsland again declined, but it was revived once again when the lake was created; the Antlers Hotel has opened as a bed-and-breakfast.

The highway through both Granite Shoals and Kingsland is lined with cafés, convenience stores, and outlets for fishing and boating supplies.

Retracing our route on FM 1431, we turned left onto FM 2342 across from the overview, driving along a slight rise of small hills and past lazy brown cattle to Park Road 4, a scenic loop curving through gently rolling land dotted with cactus and large boulders among the live oak, juniper, and mesquite trees. Shy white-tailed deer stopped and looked at us before they turned and ran away.

We learned in a hurry to be careful of the cactus thorns when we decided to stop the car by the side of the road to try to catch the deer on camera; the thorns are sharp enough to penetrate even leather shoes.

Park Road 4 leads to Inks Lake State Park and Longhorn Cavern State Park. Inks Lake State Park, centered on the smallest of the Highland Lakes, is a first-class facility with sheltered campsites along the shore. There are no camping facilities at Longhorn Cavern State Park, but there are tours of the cavern, a living cave that's still growing. The cave was a camp for Indians, a hiding place for outlaws during frontier days, a gunpowder manufacture and storage site during the Civil War, and a dance hall in the 1930s, when the folks of Burnet danced in the large Council Room. The natural air conditioning made it very popular during hot Texas summers.

According to geologists, it took a million years of water flowing through to carve out the cave, considered the largest in Texas and the third largest in the world. Although it is 11 miles long, the tour, taking an hour and a half, only covers about a mile. It's pretty cool down there, and we were glad we'd thought to bring light wraps.

From Park Road 4 we turned east onto Highway 29 along 10 miles of gently rolling green fields toward Burnet. Long white fences bordered ranches like the Granite Hills Hereford Ranch on the left, where the black-and-white cattle quietly grazed. Notice the short, feathery-leafed mesquite trees on every side, the bane of ranchers and farmers.

The Texas Legislature officially declared Burnet (pronounced BURN-it) the Bluebonnet Capital of Texas, and of course there's a big bluebonnet festival each spring. The town was established in 1849 around Fort Croghan, the third of four army forts established by the U.S. Army to protect early pioneer settlements from the Indians after the Texas Rangers moved on to other sites. Today's Fort Croghan Museum, next door to the Burnet Chamber of Commerce, has none of the original buildings still in existence, but the "Old Powder House," built during the Civil War, is joined by several stone and log buildings circa the mid-1800s that have been moved to the site. We found all sorts of relics depicting local frontier days there: restored carriages, old guns and furniture, and other exhibits.

The highway follows the tracks of the railroad that arrived in Burnet in 1882. Not long afterward, a block of the regional marble from nearby Holland quarries was shipped to Washington, D.C., as Texas's contribution to the Washington Monument.

On Burnet's historic square, one block east of the intersection of Highway 29 and U.S. 281, we browsed in the antique, arts and crafts, and other shops there.

Burnet is also the home of the Highland Lakes CAF Air Museum, headquarters for the Confederate Air Force. It's at the Burnet Municipal Airport on U.S. 281, and it has all sorts of interesting things to see, like World War II fighter planes, photographs, weapons, and other memorabilia.

Heading back on Highway 29, going west past Fort Croghan Museum and Park Road 4, we arrived at Buchanan Dam (pronounced Buck-CAN-non), which offers a spectacular view of the Highland Lakes.

The dam, dedicated in 1937, is one of the largest and oldest of its kind in the United States. A nearby building houses the Buchanan Dam Visitors Center, the Chamber of Commerce, and a museum with exhibits, old photographs, and a video about the construction of the dam. Tours of the dam are offered at certain times of the year.

The observation deck above the visitors center provides a spectacular view of both lake and dam. After we took a good look, we had fun feeding the large school of fish swimming around below the observation deck.

An entertaining side trip either before driving into Burnet or on the way to Buchanan Dam is the Vanishing Texas River Cruise. Enclosed tour boats cross Lake Buchanan into the Upper Colorado River to see wildlife and waterfalls. In summer there are dinner and sunset cruises; in winter the cruise offers a chance to view American bald eagles who nest on the banks of the river. From Highway 29 west go to FM 2341, then north about three-and-a-half miles to the dock.

The town of Buchanan Dam is located north of Highway 29, on Highway 261. It's a small resort and retirement community that grew as a result of the dam.

An interesting detour for wine buffs is a visit to Fall Creek Vineyards, north of Buchanan Dam. From the town of Buchanan Dam we drove drive north on Highway 261 to FM 2241 at Bluffton, then 2241 north to Tow. (The vineyard is about two miles northeast of Tow.) Texas is earning a fine reputation as a wine-producing state, and the winery, with

European-style buildings on the lake shore, produces Chardonnay, Chenin Blanc, sauvignon blanc, Riesling, and zinfandel. We got to sample some of the award-winning wines.

From Bluffton you have a choice of taking 2241 west through Lone Grove to Llano or returning to Highway 29 and heading west to Llano; the road is another one of the scenic routes in these parts.

Llano, which calls itself "the Deer Capital of Texas," was settled around 1855 by pioneers who had to contend with Indians stealing not only their livestock, but their clothes as well. When iron was discovered back in the late 1800s, this small town became a boomtown: Llano hoped to become "the Pittsburgh of the West." But there was none of the coal needed to turn the iron into steel, so the boom went bust and it was back to the granite business as usual. Today the streets named Bessemer and Pittsburgh remain as reminders of Llano's ambitious dream.

Then a fire destroyed much of the town north of the Llano River where most of the action took place, and all that was left was the sturdy First National Bank, now the Badu House Inn, and the old-time Bruhl's drug store, which has been restored and now houses the Llano County Museum.

Today most of Llano lies south of the river. The county courthouse was built in 1892, and a time capsule waits under a granite boulder on the west side, to be opened in the year 2056, two hundred years after the town was settled. An imposing monument to the town's Civil War dead graces the courthouse lawn.

We found that Acme Dry Goods on Main is a real nostalgia trip, an old-fashioned dry goods emporium with the original fittings still intact. The old polished-brass cash register is used to ring up sales of today's merchandise.

The Llano County Jail, built of forbidding gray granite quarried in the county, still has bars covering the arched entrance and all the windows. The original red metal roof of this Romanesque Revival building gave the jail a nickname: prisoners actually spoke fondly of "staying over at the Red Top." But if they were more serious offenders than the occasional cowboys sleeping off a night on the town, they weren't as happy with the accommodations: we climbed up the iron steps, past the dilapidated cells full of decaying cots, to the hole in the roof where the gallows swung. (The old red roof has long been replaced by a colorless metal one.) The only jailbirds today are the pigeons who come to roost through the broken upper windows and the gallows opening.

The Llano Uplift contains a treasure trove of amethysts, dolomite, garnet, quartz, and tourmaline, but unfortunately, due to the threat of lawsuits, landowners no longer feel they can permit rock hunting on their land. It is possible to find llanite, a rare brown granite embedded with crystals of pink and blue feldspar, at a cut along Highway 16 at the intersection of Highway 29, about nine or ten miles north of town. Llanite is found nowhere else in the world, so even if you're not into rock hunting, don't miss the bar in the Badu House Inn's lounge; it's made of one long slab of this famous mineral.

Packsaddle Mountain south on Highway 71 (which we viewed south of Marble Falls from that roadside park) is considered by local Llanoites to be the site in 1873 of the last Indian fight in the county. The settlers had had just about enough of the Indians helping themselves to horses, cows, and clothing, so eight of them followed a party of about twenty Apaches back to their camp atop the mountain. They killed three, and the others ran away. Descendants of the victors have marked the spot in granite on the top of the mountain, and there is also a state historical marker commemorating the event on Highway 71, fourteen miles southeast of Llano.

White-tailed deer in large numbers make Llano a center for fall deer hunters. We planned, like the deer hunters do, to be in Llano in time for a dinner of the turkey sausage that makes Inman Kitchen a restaurant famous all over the state. Barbecued beef, ham, and turkey are also delicious, along with homemade breads and pies. You won't return home hungry.

For More Information

Marble Falls/Lake LBJ Chamber of Commerce, (830) 693-4449

Bluebonnet Cafe (Marble Falls), (830) 693-2344

Antlers Hotel, (915) 388-4411 and (800) 383-0007

Inks Lake State Park (Buchanan Dam), (512) 793-2223

Longhorn Cavern State Park (Burnet), (512) 756-4680

Burnet Chamber of Commerce, (512) 756-4297

Highland Lakes CAF Air Museum, (512) 756-2226

Fort Croghan Museum (Burnet), (512) 756-8281

Vanishing Texas River Cruise (Burnet), (512) 756-6986

Lake Buchanan Chamber of Commerce (Buchanan Dam), (512) 793-2803

Fall Creek Vineyards (Tow), (915) 379-5361; in Austin call (512) 476-4477

Llano County Chamber of Commerce (Llano), (915) 247-5354

Badu House Inn (Llano), (915) 247-1207

Inman Kitchen (Llano), (915) 247-5257

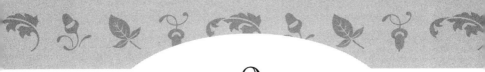

2

Texas Independence Trail

Getting there: This trip focuses on Texas Independence, making a circle from San Antonio east on U.S. 90 to Luling, south on 183 to Goliad, west on 239 to 181 to 123 to Seguin, and back to San Antonio on 90.

Highlights: Luling, the Watermelon Capital of Texas; Texas history and Palmetto State Park in Gonzales; Yorktown Pioneer Museum in an old fort; Presidio La Bahia, Mission Espiritu Santo, and the Hanging Tree in Goliad; Panna Maria, oldest Polish settlement in America; Los Nogales Museum in Seguin.

We headed east on U.S. 90 toward Luling, our mouths watering with the thought of renowned Luling barbecue for lunch. (And watermelon, too, come June.) Luling was once known as "the toughest town in Texas" (oil was discovered in 1922, and you'll probably be able to sniff the scent of oil in the air), but now it calls itself "the Watermelon Capital of Texas."

There's a Watermelon Thump every June, and juicy pink melons are on sale all summer at the farmer's market alongside the railroad tracks, but all that remains of the town's tough image is the entertaining sight of active oil wells around town, those pump jacks bobbing away even in backyards and church lawns.

Some of them are a real sight to see, like the one behind the historic log cabin of frontier preacher William Johnson in a little park on U.S. 183. It's painted like a bird, and north of the park, on the other side of U.S. 183, there's a grinning dinosaur pump jack, painted red and green.

We were ready for an early lunch at famous Old City Market Bar-B-Que, where we stood in line with the crowd for thick slabs of brisket, sausage, and white bread handed to us wrapped in pink butcher paper. Everybody just sits down at the bare wooden tables and pours on the restaurant's special sauce, either making sandwiches or eating with their fingers—primitive but finger-lickin' good.

Next we crossed Interstate 10 to State Highway 183 south to Gonzales for an interesting lesson in Texas history. But first, just after we crossed I-10 and the San Marcos River, we followed Park Road 11 on the right, leading to Palmetto State Park. The park has an amazing profusion of plants not found anywhere else in the Southwest. We stopped to marvel at the rare specimens in this botanical garden, and we weren't surprised to learn that several Texas universities use the 178-acre park as a field laboratory. Descriptive folders that interpret the nature trails are available, and the park has the usual fine camping, swimming, fishing, picnicking, and hiking facilities to be found in state parks.

After exploring the exotic foliage, we continued south to Gonzales. This town of approximately 6,500 has been called "the Lexington of Texas" because the first clash of arms in the Texas Revolution happened here. When Mexican troops demanded the town's cannon, the Texans challenged them to "come and take it!" We saw a replica of the cannon that precipitated that first skirmish.

The Gonzales Memorial Museum is a monument to that first battle and also to the 32 patriots who later answered

William Travis's call for help at the Alamo. Other historic sites are the old jail, circa 1887, complete with cells, dungeon, and gallows; Eggleston House, with antiques portraying Texas pioneer life; a Pioneer Village; and two downtown plazas, Confederate Square and Texas Heroes Square.

The St. James Inn, for rest and refreshment overnight, was built by the family of a man who made his fortune somewhat ambiguously as a "cattle gatherer" on the Chisholm Trail.

From Gonzales we took Highway 97 southwest to Cost to look at the Battle of Gonzales historical markers, then backed up a few miles to turn south on FM 108 through Smiley to FM 119 east to Yorktown, population 2,207. John York, the first settler, arrived there in 1846, unfortunately to be killed by Indians, but after a while German, Czech, and Polish immigrants settled here. Today you may hear greetings still given in those languages.

The Yorktown Pioneer Museum is housed in two separate but connected buildings, both on the National Register of Historic Places. Yorktown has three old cemeteries, Old Yorktown, Westside, and Woods Cemetery, the latter having tombstones dating from 1804.

We followed FM 119 through Weesatche ("wee" is right—all we saw of it was a sign greeting us with WELCOME TO WEESATCHE and another taking leave of us in the shape of a green four-leaf clover bearing the message AUF WEIDERSEHN) to State Highway 183 again and south about nine miles to Goliad.

Goliad is another star in the crown of Texas history. The third oldest municipality in Texas, the small town (pop. 2,000+) played a large part in the Texas Revolution. Beautiful but infamous is Presidio La Bahia, site of the Goliad Massacre. On March 26, 1836, Colonel James Fannin and his troops surrendered honorably to the

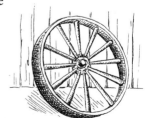

Mexicans, but were led out from imprisonment in the fort and shot, the bodies stripped and left unburied. The remains were gathered and buried three months later by General Rusk and his army. A monument now marks the gravesite, and Fannin Plaza at Market and Franklin Streets has as a centerpiece another monument, as well as four old cannons.

Goliad State Park on the edge of town is the site of beautiful Mission Espiritu Santo, built here in 1749 by the Franciscan order to convert Indians. The mission also operated a large cattle ranch.

We dined at The Empresario in the 1903 Weyland Building on the town's historic square, in sight of the Hanging Tree alongside the courthouse. But it didn't dampen our appetites: we enjoyed perusing the choices on the varied menu—seafood, steaks, grilled kabobs, and soups, sandwiches, and salads— quite a sophisticated menu for such a small town. And the lineup of homemade pies was just too tempting to resist, especially the "Sugar Free Apple Pie" and "Low Fat Chocolate Meringue Pie."

There are two country inns in Goliad, the Dial House and the Linburg House, both extremely hospitable and attractive.

Bright and early in the morning we headed west on FM 239, a Texas Independence Trail through gently rolling land, with deer crossing signs along the way but none warning of wild turkeys, which can be a hazard if they fly too close to your windshield. Jogging onto FM 72 just before Kenedy, we discovered Polak's Sawsage [sic] Farm, where Alfred and Edna Pawelek served us a delicious breakfast featuring homemade bread amid smoked Polish sausage and barbecued beef. The country store also sells homemade chowchow and other relishes and sauces. We told "Big Al" that we planned to go north on State Highway 181 to FM 123, and he cautioned, "Don't miss Panna Maria," which we wouldn't dream of doing. We were on the lookout for the famous tall white spires reaching the sky long before we turned into the settlement.

Panna Maria is the oldest Polish settlement in America, and with a population of only 96, it has done a fantastic job of putting itself on the map. Established in 1854 by Polish Catholics who named the town Virgin Mary—in Polish—they had a tough time of it, being plagued by outlaws, disease, and climate extremes they were unused to. And they were ridiculed for their foreign speech; the older generation still speaks a Silesian dialect difficult even for modern Polish speakers to understand.

Friendly folk at the visitors bureau, in a small building listed on the National Register of Historic Places, fed us iced tea and cake and told us all about their settlement. (Homemade jellies and relishes are for sale, all made by members of the town's historical society.) Then they took us on a tour of the Immaculate Conception Church, topped with a cross brought from Poland by the original colonists. The interior has an ornate altar, and there is a museum nearby, open by request.

Leaving Panna Maria reluctantly, we drove north on FM 123, and our eyes were caught almost immediately by another tall white steeple, in Cestohowa, at the intersection of FM 3191. Here the Nativity Church of Blessed Virgin Mary, built in 1873, competes for interest with a historical marker in front of the church marking the spot of El Fuerte Del Cibolo, an old Spanish fort occupied first in 1734–37 and again from 1771 to 1782. Like the church in Panna Maria, this church boasts a cross brought from Poland, in 1873.

Leaving Little Poland behind, we were back in oil country, passing farms as we drove north toward Stockdale, another tiny town that at first did not seem to have much to offer. But then we stopped at the Main Street Emporium and Tearoom, which is open seven days a week and is stocked with antiques, collectibles, and art and crafts, as well as offering lunch in the tearoom. Lunch, said proprietor Dottie Bowden when pressed to name the time, is served "anywhere from eleven to two or whatever," and she added with true small-town casualness, "and soda pop, tea, or coffee just about any time."

A surprise at the rear of the emporium was a cool room of fish tanks and fish; Lynne's Fintastics is the name.

We said goodbye to Dottie and headed north on FM 123, passing more corn and sorghum fields, as well as fine old pecan trees, on the way to Seguin. This town of 18,853 citizens was founded in 1838 as Walnut Springs by the Gonzales Rangers, but it was changed in 1839 to honor Juan N. Seguin, a distinguished Mexican-Texan who served in Sam Houston's Army of Texas Independence. We saw many pre-Texas Revolution buildings here, designated by historical markers.

Among them we found the Magnolia Hotel of 1824 and the Juan Seguin Post Office, built by the Mexican government in 1823. The one-room adobe structure now houses Los Nogales Museum, with Texas historical papers, pictures, and furniture. We were pleasantly puzzled by a tiny white-painted Victorian house to the left of Los Nogales, small enough to be a dollhouse or playhouse. "That's what it is," we were told, "the last thing built by a local toy maker." It sure is cute.

Around the corner we found the Campbell Log Cabin, built in 1850 and moved to this location, furnished, and open to tourists, and on Courthouse Square we were amazed to discover the "World's Largest Pecan," a two-and-a-half-foot-long nut made of metal and plaster and set in solid cement, a tribute to the official Texas state tree.

For More Information

Luling Area Chamber of Commerce, (830) 875-3214

Palmetto State Park, (830) 672-3266

Gonzales Chamber of Commerce, (830) 672-6533

St. James Inn (Gonzales), (830) 672-7066

Goliad Chamber of Commerce, (512) 645-3563

Goliad State Park, (512) 645-3405

Empresario Restaurant (Goliad), (512) 645-2347

Dial House, (512) 645-3366

Linburg House, (512) 645-1997

Polak's Sawsage Farm (Karnes City), (830) 583-2113

Panna Maria Visitor Center, (830) 780-4471

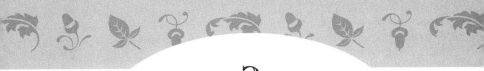

3

Texas Hill Country Trail I

Getting there: This trip focuses on the northern half of the beautiful Texas Hill Country. From Austin, take I-35 south to FM 150 at Kyle and go west through Kyle. You will return to Austin on Highway 290 east.

Highlights: Katherine Anne Porter's girlhood home in Kyle; Wimberley antique shops; quaint Blanco; funny Luckenbach; Lyndon B. Johnson's birthplace and the LBJ Ranch in Stonewall; historic Fredericksburg; Enchanted Rock; Johnson City; and Pedernales Falls State Park.

The Texas Hill Country (geologically the Edwards Plateau) is known for winding, curving roads and panoramic vistas over wooded hills green with pin oak, cedar, mesquite, and cactus. In spring, the fields are carpeted with bluebonnets and Indian Paintbrush. This northern part of the Hill Country is sort of an in-between place, with softer, humid lands to the east, and stretching to the west toward high plains, plateaus, and deserts. Small valleys contain scattered farms and ranches where fat cattle graze among the rocks and cedar. Many farmhouses and other buildings are built of the local limestone, rocks pried from the soil and blocks quarried from the hills. Oak and mesquite line the roads, and every once in a while cactus, either yucca or prickly pear, appears in the underbrush amid the rocks.

Sheep graze among the cattle, and there are no billboards or signs of any kind for miles and miles. In fact, "if you ignore the telephone and power lines along the way, there'd be nothing," said my traveling companion. But I was too busy admiring the wooded hills, broad ranchlands, and wide vistas to reply.

From Austin via Interstate 35 south, we took the exit for Kyle, FM 150, and drove west down Center Street, the main thoroughfare of this small town. We wanted to take a look at the white frame house on the corner of Sledge and Center (facing the Baptist Church), which was the girlhood home of writer Katherine Anne Porter. Now a museum, the historic house, built in 1880, is furnished with period pieces, as well as a collection of pictures and writings. The museum has a growing collection of works by Southwest writers, artists, and poets.

The author of such works as *Ship of Fools* was raised by her grandmother, and the stone "upping block" used to mount horses is still in the front yard. In the nearby cemetery you can find Porter's grandparents' graves, an old hanging tree, and the slave cemetery. The museum also has a collection of tools, weapons, and artwork, relics of Native Americans who lived in the area for some 40,000 years.

Leaving Kyle and the museum behind us, we followed FM 150 to FM 3237 to the small unincorporated village of Wimberley. Many Wimberley residents are descendants of the pioneers of 1848, which is when William Calvin Winters built a mill on the creek. In 1872 Pleasant Wimberley bought the mill, and the village ended up being named for him. The day we were there the whole area was bustling, since this was one of the Lion's Market Days (first Saturday, April through September), the best time to shop for antiques, collectibles, and crafts.

Crossing Cypress Creek, we passed an intriguing sign—IN SEASON, APPLES AND PEACHES, YOU PICK 'EM—and shot right from the bridge into the Village Square, a pie-shaped wedge lined with shops, restaurants, and galleries year-round. We found Wimberley quaint, pretty, friendly, and only crowded on market days!

Leaving Wimberley, we headed northwest on FM 2325 to FM 165 along the calm green waters of the Blanco River toward Blanco. We passed a low dam where kids were having fun, balancing across it. The river banks were lined neatly with concrete overhung with green shrubbery. We noticed many small dams as we went along; flash floods are a real danger here. There are so many low dips and roller-coaster spots in the Hill Country roads that you want to be sure to pay attention to the high-water gauges and the signs along the way warning: STREAM CROSSINGS SUBJECT TO FLOODING IN WET WEATHER. Since the river winds, we crossed it once again as we passed into town, and we spotted an old cemetery on our left.

Blanco was settled in 1853 by pioneer stockmen who shouldn't have been surprised when they found they had to fortify their homes against hostile Indians. The town was the county seat from 1858 to 1891, and we were told that the stone Blanco County Courthouse in the center of town is an example of Second Empire–style architecture. Now the county seat is in Johnson City, further proof that this area owes much of its fame to the late president Lyndon B. Johnson.

Blanco Town Hall and small shops face the courthouse on the square. The Pecan Street Bakery and Cafe looked tempting, but it was too early for lunch, so we popped into Strickland Drugs to see if by lucky chance they still had an old-fashioned soda fountain. Instead we found, amid the modern items, a glass display case containing all sorts of old-fashioned jars and bottles. "The man who bought the store, he found all that old medicine out back," the clerk told us; it was an interesting collection.

The square's two-block City Park joins Blanco State Park, which lies within the city limits along scenic Blanco River Valley. The 110-acre park has camping, trailer sites, picnicking, screened shelters, a group pavilion, and offers fishing, swimming, pedal boats, and a children's play area in addition to restrooms and showers.

There's a Town Creek Nature Trail in Roland and Viola Bindseil Park, and for a particularly scenic drive along the ridge called the Devil's Backbone, we drove south on FM 32 two miles to enjoy the view. Then we retraced our route back to Blanco and took FM 1623 to Stonewall, famed equally for delicious Gillespie County peaches and LBJ Ranch, late president Lyndon B. Johnson's home.

Stonewall, named for Confederate General Stonewall Jackson, was founded in 1870. At Lyndon B. Johnson State Park and LBJ National Historic Site east of town, we joined the laughing crowd listening to recordings of LBJ's jokes before boarding a small tour bus around the ranch to see LBJ's birthplace, his one-room schoolhouse, and other historic sites.

Full of recent history, we headed west on Highway 290 for a taste of older Texas history in Fredericksburg, where natives still speak German and live in quaint gingerbread-trimmed houses. But first we took a little detour south on FM 1376 for four miles to Luckenbach, famed in song and story.

Luckenbach was founded in 1849 but it never amounted to anything and was a ghost town by the 1970s. Nobody would have heard of Luckenbach if the late storyteller of Texas folklore, Hondo Crouch, hadn't bought the town in 1970. It was brought to further notoriety by country-western stars Willie Nelson and Waylon Jennings; the latter recorded the song

"Luckenbach, Texas," and they both sang it. Such is fame that the few events held there became news, so naturally we were curious.

Crouch had a reputation as a humorist, and the joke was evident when we arrived: the "town" consists of an unpainted wooden general store and one or two other structures that sometimes are revived as dance hall and beer tavern. The bend in the road is marked by homemade VISIT UPTOWN LUCKEN-BACH signs (the highway department gave up trying to mark the spot officially; the signs were stolen faster than they were posted). You'd be smart to call the General Store before arriving to find out whether anything's happening—nothing was while we were there! (But the store hands out free postcards with charming pen-and-ink sketches to illustrate that there's nothing much to photograph!)

Almost running over a glistening wet armadillo who was taking his time crossing the road, we retraced our route back to Highway 290 toward Fredericksburg, where a great deal was happening. Walking through the historic district, we were struck by the number of historical markers; the town was settled in 1846 by immigrant families from Germany, and their leader, John Meusebach, established lasting peace with the surrounding Commanches a year later.

These days one of Fredericksburg's big celebrations is the Easter Fires, commemorating the peace talks. While the Indians and settlers were sitting around fires awaiting the outcome of the peace talks, a pioneer mother quieted her children's fears by telling them a charming tale of the Easter rabbit who lit and tended those hillside fires to boil the traditional eggs. Today, hillside fires glow each Easter eve while a pageant retells the story.

Possibly unique to Fredericksburg are the Sunday Houses, tiny homes built by early settlers to use on weekends. From farms and ranches miles away they would journey into town and stay in these small houses for Saturday marketing (and polka-ing) and Sunday church. Although the ones left are private residences, open only for occasional tours, we enjoyed driving by and taking a look. (Some now serve as bed-and-breakfast establishments.)

A particular point of interest is the Admiral Nimitz Museum in the Nimitz Steamboat Hotel. Nimitz was born here, and the hotel belonged to his grandfather. We wondered what had inspired the World War II admiral to join the navy, since the largest body of water anywhere around here is the Pedernales River! Behind the hotel, an open-air History Walk displays guns, boats, and planes from World War II along the pathways. Particularly lovely is the Japanese Garden of Peace, a gift from the people of Japan.

Speaking of quaint, the Vereins Kirche Museum building is something to see: the eight-sided structure looks just like a giant coffee mill. It was the first public building in the town, serving as a house of worship, school, and meeting hall. Now it holds city archives, a local history collection, and archaeological items.

After a fulsome meal of sauerbraten and strudel at George's Old German Bakery and Cafe on Main Street, we headed north on Ranch Road 965 to Enchanted Rock. (Fredericksburg has dozens of bed-and-breakfast inns if you want to spend the night and see even more of this historic spot.)

We were wearing the right shoes to climb this round pink "granite" mound, considered among the oldest (one billion years) exposed rocks in North America, rising like a huge bald pate above the 1,643-acre park. Myriad tales and legends have contributed to the name "enchanted."

Occasionally catching sight of deer, we continued north on RR 965, turned right on FM 16, and followed it south to 1323, which led us to Johnson City and some more LBJ history. The town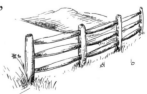

is named for the pioneer Johnson family, ancestors of the president. Long before he was born, his grandfather Sam Ealy Johnson, Sr., with Sam's brother Tom ran a cattle empire here back when Texas was still open range. They rounded up longhorns and drove them up the Chisholm Trail in the 1860s.

In Johnson City's Lyndon B. Johnson National Historic Park (don't get mixed up with the LBJ Ranch and State Park 14 miles west in Stonewall) we saw the white frame, white picket-fenced boyhood home of the president, a far cry from the rustic farmhouse he was born in in Stonewall. A block west we found Johnson's Settlement, the old ranch complex owned by the president's grandfather and great-uncle from 1867 to 1872. It was a gathering point for seven counties for cattle drives.

The settlement also served as an aid station for those wounded in the Deer Creek Indian Battle. An original "dog run," cabin, barn, and other buildings are restored and are part of the "living history" program offered by the park.

(Johnson City has joined the trend for bed-and-breakfast places with small, two-guest-room cottages. The town is a nice, relaxing place to spend the night, and Carolyn's Cottage was pretty cute.)

Crossing Highway 281 onto FM 2766, we drove east to Pedernales Falls State Park, 4,800 scenic acres preserving the natural Hill Country beauty of the area, with panoramic views over the hills. In a good rainfall year the waterfalls on the Pedernales River here are pretty picturesque, and the park has abundant plant and animal life.

FM 2766 ends at the park, but FM 3232 leads south just outside the entrance, and we passed more Hill Country panoramic views as we drove toward Highway 290 to head east to Austin. On the way, two baby deer, bold as you please, stopped in the middle of the highway and glared at us as though we were the interlopers. We had to honk the horn several times to get them to move; it wasn't until the third honk that they turned and gracefully bounded back into the underbrush alongside the road.

For More Information

Katherine Anne Porter Museum, (512) 268-2220

Wimberley Chamber of Commerce, (512) 847-2201

Blanco Chamber of Commerce, (830) 833-5101

Stonewall Chamber of Commerce, (830) 644-2735

LBJ State Park and LBJ National Historical Site (Stonewall), (830) 644-2252

Luckenbach General Store, (830) 997-3224

Fredericksburg Convention & Visitors Bureau, (830) 997-6523

Admiral Nimitz State Historical Park (Fredericksburg), (830) 997-4379

Vereins Kirche Museum (Fredericksburg), (830) 997-7832 or (830) 997-2835

Bed and Breakfast Reservation Services of Fredericksburg, (830) 997-4712

Enchanted Rock State Natural Area, (915) 247-3903

LBJ National Historic Park (Johnson City), (830) 868-7128

Johnson City Bed and Breakfast Association, (830) 868-4548

Pedernales Falls State Park, (830) 868-7304

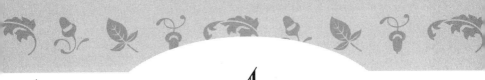

4

Texas Hill Country Trail II

Getting there: This trip focuses on the southern half of the beautiful Texas Hill Country. From San Antonio, take I-35 north past New Braunfels to FM 306 west to Sattler. You will return to San Antonio on Highway 90 east.

Highlights: Sattler and dinosaur tracks; Canyon Lake and Natural Bridge Caverns; Guadalupe River State Park; Boerne and Cave Without a Name; Camp Verde; Kerrville, Ingram, and Hunt on the Guadalupe; Utopia and the Sabinal River; Hondo with dinosaur tracks; and the Alsatian settlement of Castroville.

Rugged Edwards Plateau, otherwise known as the Hill Country, is famous for winding, curving roads and panoramic vistas over wooded hills green with pin oak, cedar, mesquite, and cactus. It is also threaded with caves and caverns, especially in the southern part. In this rocky land, buildings small and large are constructed of Hill Country rocks, more manageable-sized ones pried from the soil rather than the large blocks of limestone quarried to the north. As you head south, oak gives way to cedar and mesquite, and the rolling hills and panoramic views are more pronounced. The area is laced with cool green rivers, providing soothing coolness to this relatively high, arid land.

Driving the country roads in summertime, you'll see both children and grownups cavorting in the cool water along the small dams built to control the waters during spring floods. Flash floods are a real danger here; pay attention to the high water gauges and the signs along the roads.

We drove north on I-35 to FM 306 just a few miles north of New Braunfels, then headed west on FM 306 fourteen miles to FM 2673 to Sattler, nestled in the rolling Hill Country. While Sattler (recent population count 30) is mainly a center for all the activity around Canyon Lake, we wanted to see Dinosaur Flats, where hundreds of dinosaur tracks were uncovered by excavators in 1982. In the long-ago limey mud of a saltwater marsh by an ancient sea, three-toed and round-footed "thunder lizards" walked. Eventually the mud turned into limestone, preserving all those dinosaur tracks.

Canyon Lake is worth a stop, too. Just continue west on FM 306 to see one of the most scenic lakes in Texas. The 8,240-acre lake, built by the U.S. Army Corps of Engineers, is spread among steep-banked, evergreen hills and offers anything and everything in the way of water sports and enjoyment: fishing, boating, swimming, camping, picnicking, and spectacular fishing. The record for catfish is 86 pounds; for striped bass 25.5 pounds. That's a lot of fish!

But this wasn't a fishing trip, so we retraced our route through Sattler and down FM 2673 to FM 2722 to Highway 46. We wanted to visit the vaunted Natural Bridge Caverns, so we turned south off Highway 46 onto FM 1863 to the caverns, a vast subterranean maze designated as a U.S. Natural Landmark. Here we walked beneath a natural rock bridge (hence the name) into the hillside and down through long cool underground corridors. For about a mile we strolled through giant rooms with awesome cave formations, all leading to underground Purgatory Creek. The stalagmites and stalactites were fantastic, and we had to blink when we came out into the sunshine again.

Again retracing our route back to Highway 46, we continued west, crossing Highway 281 and heading for Boerne. This is lovely scenic Hill Country land, with curving, hilly roads, and once in a while a quick glimpse of deer. Along the way, we passed Guadalupe River State Park on our right. The scenic park is bisected by the cypress-edged banks of the river. On the far side of the river are magnificent limestone cliffs; wildlife within the park includes white-tailed deer, coyotes, foxes, and armadillos. Bird-watchers can spot the rare golden-cheeked warbler. "If they're lucky," my traveling companion said—but they do nest there in the juniper thickets.

Boerne (pronounced BURR-nee) began in 1849 as a village called Tusculum. It was renamed by German pioneers in 1851, honoring a German political writer. Boerne has a cave, too, Cave Without a Name, and we drove up FM 474 to see

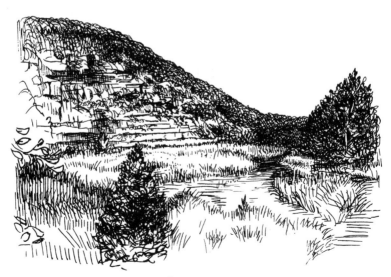

Guadalupe River State Park

it. Like everyone else, we asked, "Why no name?" Seems that when the cave was discovered and opened in 1939, a contest was held to name it. The contest was won by a young boy who said, "This cave is too pretty to name." That turned out to be true; the cave, 98 percent of which is still accessible, has huge cavernous rooms with the most fantastically imaginative formations hanging from the roofs (too high to call ceilings) and growing from the walls.

Wonderful as both the caves were, we were a little caved out, so we went to check out Ye Kendall Inn, Boerne's stage-coach stop built in 1859 on an unusually large green square, grounds for festivals and fairs. The inn was a gathering place for Texas lawmen, army officers, cattle drovers, and other frontier characters; the high windows in the back look suspiciously like openings for rifles. There's a rumor that an old secret tunnel runs from the inn to a building on the corner of the square. We couldn't find out about that, but we found delicious food in the restaurant, chic shopping in the lobby/boutique, and fine accommodations in the guest rooms upstairs and off the back patio.

From Boerne, we continued west on Highway 46 to Highway 16, where we turned north through steep hills of scenery through Pipe Creek and on to Bandera. (There was a flea market going on in Pipe Creek, but my companion wouldn't stop!) Bandera bills itself the "Cowboy Capital of the World." It was founded in 1852 as a cypress shingle camp, and a Mormon colony was established here in 1854. Today, Bandera, on beautiful cool and clear Medina River, is surrounded by dude ranches. The town offers western activities, too, from rugged rodeos to country-western music and dancing, downtown at Arky Blue's Silver Dollar Saloon (among others). There's even parimutuel betting at Bandera Downs, both thoroughbred and quarter horse races.

But Bandera earns its cowboy capital title mostly because it's an authentic western town, surrounded by working as well as guest ranches. The wranglers who take dudes out on the trail are the real thing; they drive and rope cattle the rest of the time.

From Bandera we went north on FM 173 to Camp Verde, a sort of Texas joke. After Texas joined the Union, the U.S. Army established a chain of forts along the frontier to protect settlers. One of these outposts was Camp Verde on Verde Creek, and this camp had the dubious distinction of being the only camel base on the frontier.

Camel? Yep. Jefferson Davis, Secretary of War in 1855, had the bright idea of purchasing a herd of camels to study whether they would make better pack animals in the West than horses and mules. This interesting experiment was interrupted by the Civil War, and reports say that by the time the war was over, the camels were scattered all over. The experiment was not resumed, probably because by then the railroads were beginning to replace pack animals of all kinds.

The army abandoned the camp in 1869, and we found there's not much left of Camp Verde except the Camp Verde General Store. But it's a fine old-timey store, and the friendly folks there enjoy telling the tale of the Texas camels.

Heading north, we reached Highway 16 again just below Kerrville and crossed the Guadalupe River into town. Kerrville is one of Texas's most popular health and recreation centers, with more than two dozen boys' and girls' summer camps along the beautiful clear river. An early settler, Charles Schreiner, a native of France, served with the Confederacy as a captain, then as a Texas Ranger, and ended up establishing a general merchandising business in Kerrville in 1869. We saw the Schreiner name all over town.

We looked at some wonderful works in the Cowboy Artists of America Museum, a splendid showcase for contemporary cowboy artists. The handsome Romanesque stone Hill Country Museum, former home of Captain Schreiner, contains antiques, artifacts, and memorabilia from the region.

Then it was time to head west again, this time on Highway 39 along the Guadalupe toward Ingram and Hunt, recreational communities on the river. At the intersection of Highway 27 in Ingram, we caught a glimpse of some huge murals painted on a long building on the right side of the road. I hollered "Whoa!" We turned back to see the Kerr County Historical Murals, "History on a Wall," painted and installed on the T. J. Moore Lumber Company building.

Continuing along 39, we followed the tree-shaded banks of the Guadalupe River, past parks and summer camps. The road wound around past peach orchards—the trees thrive in the rocky soil—and over one-lane bridges crossing the South Fork of the Guadalupe, which just wouldn't quit. The river was so tempting that we stopped and went wading for a little while, and the water was so cool and refreshing that we put our shoes and socks back on reluctantly.

But we wanted to see the famous lost maples, so on we went until we reached FM 187. There we turned south where the road begins to climb down from the 2,300-foot-high Edwards Plateau. Sinkholes, the porous basins that feed rainwater into the deep Edwards Aquifer, dot the Hill Country, and we saw a good example on the west edge of 187 about 10 miles south of Highway 39.

The road led along the Sabinal River to Vanderpool, which has a recorded population of only 20 but is significant as the site of the famous Lost Maples State Natural Area.

The maples aren't really lost, they're just unusual for Texas—thriving in small, protected pockets where humidity is moderate and moisture is retained. The leaves turn brilliant yellow and orange in the fall—a welcome sight in a state where just about nothing else does. Again, as in Guadalupe River State Park, lucky bird-watchers might catch glimpses of that elusive golden-cheeked warbler. We didn't.

From Lost Maples we turned west onto one of the most spectacular roads in the Hill Country, FM 337, where massive wooded steeps surround tiny hidden valleys and the road makes some hairpin curves and roller-coaster dips.

Crossing the Frio River, we came to Leakey (pronounced LAY-key), one of the most scenic, picturesque areas of the Hill Country. Here, elevations range from 1,500 to 2,400 feet, with dramatic canyons cut into the rock by the Frio and Nueces Rivers. Archaeologists have found evidence of prehistoric civilizations here, and at the time of the Spanish explorers this was Comanche and Apache land.

Driving south from Leakey on Highway 83, we couldn't resist turning east and crossing back over the Frio River on FM 1050 because we wanted to drive back through the wonderful scenery we enjoyed on FM 337. Besides, it was only 10 miles to Utopia, and who could resist taking a look at a place with a name like that?

Well, you guessed it, Utopia's not very big, but it's a lovely out-of-the-way place on the Sabinal River. An early postmaster read Sir Thomas Moore's description of Utopia and got carried away, figuring he'd found the perfect place described by Moore: perfect climate and perfect, happy people. And we were two happy, if perhaps not perfect, people after a delicious chicken-fried steak dinner at Utopia's Lost Maples Cafe.

A good resting place is Utopia on the River, a resort on lovely grounds beside the Sabinal River, among pecan and mesquite trees. Next, we took FM 470 east through some more spectacular Hill Country scenery—dramatic blue hills surrounding small green valleys, with sparkling rivers and creeks threading through. Those roller-coaster roads with hairpin curves sure kept us awake and alert!

At Tarpley we turned south on FM 462 toward Hondo to see more dinosaur tracks. They're embedded in Hondo Creek about 23 miles north of Hondo, and are easily seen. Preserved in stone, they were made by herb-eating trachodons, dinosaurs about 40 feet long.

By now we'd come to Highway 90, and we headed east for San Antonio. But we couldn't resist stopping at Castroville on the way. This "Little Alsace of Texas" was founded in 1844 by Henri Castro, who brought his group of Alsatian settlers to Texas and parked them along a picturesque curve of the Medina River.

Landmark Inn, a state historic structure, served as rest stop for stagecoach travelers back then. Restored in the 1940s, the inn is in business again, and it is a treat to go back in time, sitting and rocking on the gallery and contemplating the old water-powered gristmill on the river. There's a huge oak tree by the river, too, and legend has it that Geronimo spent a night tied to it while his captors took it easy at the inn.

From Castroville it was a mere 39 miles east on Highway 90 back to San Antonio.

For More Information

Canyon Lake Chamber of Commerce, (830) 964-2223 or (800) 528-2104

Natural Bridge Caverns, (830) 651-6101

Guadalupe River State Park, (830) 438-2656

Boerne Chamber of Commerce, (830) 249-8000

Cave Without a Name (Boerne), (830) 537-4212

Ye Kendall Inn (Boerne), (830) 249-2138 and (800) 364-2138

Bandera Convention & Visitors Bureau, (210) 796-3045 or (800) 364-3833

Kerrville Area Chamber of Commerce, (210) 896-1155

West Kerr County Chamber of Commerce (Ingram and Hunt), (830) 367-4322 or (800) 257-4322

Lost Maples State Natural Area, (830) 966-3413

Lost Maples Cafe (Utopia) (830) 966-2221

Utopia on the River, (830) 966-2444

Castroville Chamber of Commerce, (210) 538-3142

Landmark Inn, (830) 931-2133 (reservations: (512) 389-8900)

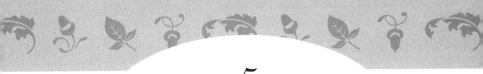

5

East Texas Trail I

Getting there: This trip focuses on the Davy Crockett National Forest area, beginning in Tyler, making a circle around the forest, and visiting historical towns surrounding the forest. From Tyler take Highway 110 south to Rusk, about 60 miles. You'll return to Tyler on FM 315 north to Highway 31 east.

Highlights: Texas Forest Trails through beautiful East Texas Piney Woods; Davy Crockett National Forest; Rusk with Jim Hogg State Historical Park and Texas State Railroad; Millard's Crossing and other attractions in Nacogdoches; Alto and prehistoric Caddoan Mounds; Crockett, where acccording to legend Davy camped on the way to meet his fate at the Alamo; and Palestine, with Davey Dogwood Park.

We left Tyler bright and early, knowing we had a lot of history to cover, from prehistoric Indians to Alamo hero Davy Crockett, as well as a great deal of scenic country roads amid the famed East Texas Piney Woods. Heading south on Highway 110, we drove through Whitehouse and across Mud Creek to Troup. The highway went through town, past Troup's old-fashioned and weathered downtown stores, then turned east into a much prettier country road. We drove through the tiny settlement of Black Jack toward New Sum-

37

merfield beneath a shady green canopy of tall Texas pines. After a while, the road led past open fields, and on our right we passed what seemed like hundreds of plastic-covered mounds. Finally the mystery was solved: the mounds turned out to be the greenhouses of a huge wholesale nursery!

Crossing Highway 79 at New Summerfield, we drove past a large cemetery on the right; to the left, far vistas of rolling green land stood as a contrast to the dense growths of pine we'd been passing through.

Coming into Rusk, named for Thomas Jefferson Rusk, a signer of the Texas Declaration of Independence, we headed for Footbridge Garden Park. We were curious to see the 546-foot bridge, said to be the nation's longest. It was built in 1861 for crossing the valley during the rainy season; now the wooded setting is a lovely park.

Also of interest was the Old Rusk Penitentiary Building, main building of the former Rusk State Prison, built in 1878. Prisoners here made the iron dome of the State Capitol in Austin (which we're told is seven feet higher than the nation's Capitol in Washington, D.C.!).

South of town, we headed west on Highway 84 to see the site of the Texas State Railroad at Rusk/Palestine State Park, a one-hundred-acre park amid towering pines. The antique steam-powered passenger train is operated by the Texas Parks and Wildlife Department and runs through the longest, skinniest state park in the country. Choo-chooing through incredibly dense forest land, the train travels 25.5 miles west to Palestine, and since we knew that Palestine was on our return route to Tyler, it was tempting to hop aboard. But then, we were on a driving trip—and what would we do with the car?

So we reserved that fun train trip for another day and turned back on Highway 84 northeast to the Jim Hogg State Historical Park. James Stephen Hogg was the first native-born Texan to serve as governor, and the 175-acre scenic forest of lofty pines is dedicated as a memorial to him. Leaving the park, we continued east on Highway 84. Crossing Highway 69, we caught a surprising glimpse, on the left side of the road, of some emus. (An emu farm? But my driver wouldn't stop!) Leaving Highway 84, we turned on to FM 343 toward Nacogdoches. This was a wonderful road, hilly and curvy with lots of long downhill roller-coaster runs. We passed an amazing number of mobile homes settled comfortably into the pines— one even had a beautifully trimmed privet hedge set around it.

We drove under the high overpass of Highway 59, and just beyond that we took Business 59, designated a Texas Forest Trail, into Nacogdoches.

Nacogdoches was the site of an Indian settlement long before Europeans arrived on the scene, and the town is named for those Indians. La Salle happened by when he was in the area; a Spanish mission was founded in 1716. Locals claim that North Street, which began life as "La Calle del Norte," is the oldest public thoroughfare in the United States.

There's too much here to see in just a day (there are several good bed-and-breakfast inns—Mound Street Inn, Haden Edwards Inn, and the Hardeman Guest House, if you want to spend the night). Don't miss Millard's Crossing, a group of restored 19th-century log cabins and wooden buildings furnished with antiques and pioneer memorabilia. The Old Stone Fort was built in 1779 as a Spanish trading post, and later it hosted four unsuccessful attempts to establish the Republic of Texas. There's a lovely garden of native and exotic trees, shrubs, and vines at the Stephen F. Austin Arboretum & Herb Garden on the campus of Stephen F. Austin University.

But "Enough!" cried my chauffeur, so we saved more for another day and headed west on Highway 21 for the small town of Alto. At first hilly with curves, the road flattened out into a landscape of grasslands loaded with grazing cattle. Alto was named Spanish for "high" because it's the highest point between the Angelina and Neches Rivers, and there was a sure-enough cool breeze from atop the hills.

We continued west on Highway 21 toward Crockett, along the north edge of Davy Crockett National Forest, which encompasses 161,500 acres of the heavily forested Piney Woods. Here the highway changed to a flat straight road. (An alternate route is Highway 7, which goes smack through the center of the forest to Crockett, but we continued west on Highway 21 because we wanted to visit Caddoan Mounds State Historic Site. We did stop at the Neches Bluff Overlook, seven miles southwest into the park, for a magnificent view.) We found Caddoan Mounds on Highway 21, six miles west of Alto.

Caddoan Mounds is an important archaeological spot in Texas. Evidence points to occupation by Early Caddo Indians around A.D. 800–1300, and closer analysis reveals earlier occupations by Paleoindian (10,000–6,000 B.C.) and Archaic (6,000 B.C.–A.D. 500) cultures. We found a full-size replica of a Caddoan house (built with Stone Age tools) as well as a visitors center and an interpretive trail. Two ceremonial mounds 300 by 350 feet still remain from the ancient Indian culture; they are now covered with grass and don't look like much. Wonder what they contain? If an archaeological excavation is in progress, we were told, visitors are welcome to observe and ask questions, but we weren't lucky enough to be there at the right time.

Leaving the site, we crossed the Neches River and passed endless historical markers, one of which pointed to a "Pepper Tree planted in 1848." There were so many my driver became very amused. "If you stopped and looked at them all, you'd never get out of here" was his opinion. So we didn't stop for any since we were eager to reach Crockett, by way of Weches.

Weches is a tiny community (population 26) first settled in 1847 on the northern boundary of Davy Crockett National Forest. It was established on the site of a Spanish mission that had been established in 1690, 150 years earlier, at a large Tejas

Indian village nearby. Mission Tejas State Historic Park, two miles southwest of Weches, commemorates the Mission San Francisco de los Tejas. It was not successful and it closed but opened again in 1716 to stem a French settlement. When the French threat never materialized, the mission moved to San Antonio in 1731.

The park also contains a log stagecoach stop, home of the Rice family and one of many such along El Camino Real (the Royal Highway, which linked Mexico City with Sante Fe from the sixteenth to the nineteenth century). Hostile Indians caused the family to abandon the site, but eventually they returned.

Crockett, obviously, is named for Davy Crockett, one of the heroes who died at the Alamo. Almost everything in town is named for Davy: in addition to the forest there's Davy Crockett Memorial Park and Davy Crockett Spring, which is said to be the campsite of the small detachment of men headed for San Antonio and the Alamo. But we also visited the Monroe-Crook House, an elegant 1854 home with period furnishings, and the Downs-Aldrich House, a restored three-story Victorian gingerbread mansion circa 1891. (Warfield House, built around 1897, is now a lovely bed-and-breakfast surrounded by a wraparound porch and shaded by pecan trees.)

From Crockett we went north on FM 2022, a gently rolling wooded and curving drive through dense trees with no road signs or billboards except for a small roadside stand on the left offering yams for sale and another on the right touting farm-fresh eggs. This was a pretty country road, winding along what we decided must be an overgrown Christmas tree farm, since there were so many just the right shape (but much too large for the living room!).

At one point my chauffeur hollered "Look at that big black snake!" but I missed it—he drives kind of fast. (We also passed quite a few dead armadillos along the way; the slow creatures are the butt of many a Texas joke about roadkill, which I doubt would be funny to the poor animals if they could understand them.)

FM 2022 ended at Highway 234, and we jogged along it to Slocum, where we began to pass oil pump jacks working away amid the grazing cows. One was pumping away right out in front of Strong's Memorial Cemetery, and another on the pasture just beyond. Heading north to FM 2419, we passed a lot more amid the hay and feed lots, although we rarely saw another car going either way.

Farmhouses were scattered here and there as the road became slightly more hilly, and we passed another pretty cemetery at Walton Springs.

FM 2419 ended suddenly at Highway 287, and we drove four miles north into Palestine (which in Texas is pronounced PAL-es-teen.) We'd arrived at the other end of the Texas State Railroad, which we'd been tempted to take in Rusk. The terminal is four miles east on Highway 84 at the state park.

Davey Dogwood Park just north of town is a four-hundred-acre spot of picturesque rolling hills, clear streams, forest, and meadow—especially famous in spring for the flowering dogwood trees. (There's an annual Texas Dogwood Trail in late March or early April, depending on when the trees bloom.)

Palestine has an Old Magnolia Frontier Town, whose historic buildings have been assembled to re-create a 19th-century Old West town. Two museums, the Palestine Firefighters' (this is forest country, remember) and the Museum for East Texas Culture, are interesting. The latter is housed in an old 1915 schoolhouse (1915 is old for Texas).

From Palestine we took FM 315, a Texas Forest Trail, north through Poyner around some nice curves along cattle ranches and a little white Baptist church on the left. Past Poyner, the road became hilly and curving, with a hairpin curve or two. The road turned into a sort of causeway as it crossed beautiful blue Lake Palestine—the only flaw we saw (and it could be a big one to boaters) was hundreds of dry tree stumps and branches poking up out of the water.

An amusing sight on the other side of the lake was a farmhouse gate with two geese perched on top of the gateposts—perhaps a change, we guessed, from the newly repopular pink flamingos.

Hungry, we stopped at Nate's Place, a half-mile north of the lake, where we were greeted with a "howdy" as though we were just two more of the regulars enjoying a bite in the café half of the general store. The barbecued beef, potato salad, and cole slaw, served in baskets on the oilcloth tablecloths, tasted delicious, and the Big Red soda pop was the perfect accompaniment. And just count the homemade pies: apple, chocolate, lemon, coconut, pecan, Hawaiian dessert, buttermilk, and egg custard. We couldn't make a decision, so we abstained, good for the waistline.

The friendly waitresses did double duty as cashiers for the store half of Nate's Place, and while waiting to pay the check, we wandered around looking at the interesting merchandise. I was puzzling over some strange transparent rubbery green and red things shaped like worms and tadpoles that looked alarmingly like a kind of candy I've only seen before in fruit shapes and colors, when waitress-cashier Kathy assured me, "Oh that, it's just bait for fishing."

Happily stuffed, we headed north again along FM 315 and turned east on Highway 31 back to Tyler.

For More Information

Tyler Chamber of Commerce, (903) 592-1661

Rusk Chamber of Commerce, (903) 683-4242

Texas State Railroad, (800) 442-8951

Nacogdoches Convention and Visitors Bureau, (409) 564-7351

Mound Street Inn (Nacogdoches), (409) 569-2211

Haden Edwards Inn (Nacogdoches), (409) 564-9999

Hardeman Guest House (Nacogdoches), (409) 569-1947

Caddoan Mounds State Historical Park , (409) 858-3218

Mission Tejas State Historic Site, (409) 687-2394

Warfield House (Crockett), (409) 544-4037

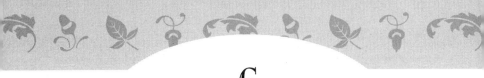

6

East Texas Trail II

Getting there: This trip focuses on northeast Texas: forest trails, lakes, and antiques galore. From Longview take Highway 80 west to Gladewater. You'll return to Longview on I-20 west (and on to Dallas on I-20 west).

Highlights: Gladewater antiques; Mineola boutiques; Quitman history; Winnsboro charm; Pittsburg antiques and fruit; Lake O' the Pines; historic Jefferson; Caddo Lake; Karnack, Lady Bird Johnson's birthplace; Marshall and pottery.

From Longview we took Highway 80 thirteen short miles west to Gladewater, which enjoys the title of "Antique Capital of East Texas." Whether you're into antiques or not, you won't be able to resist registering amazement at the many shops lining the main street of this small town (pop. 6,000+). We began to feel that the number of shops outnumbered the citizens! (Actually, there are about two dozen antique and crafts shops—it just seemed like more, seeing them all in a row on the main street and around the corners.)

When the Texas and Pacific Railroad was built here in 1872, the residents of a small community named St. Claire, a few miles to the east, moved over en masse to benefit from the new railway. Then when oil was discovered in 1931, the population grew again, doubling overnight until it reached 100,000 at the height of the boom. We went to examine the derrick and pumping unit preserved in the 100 block of West Commerce: the historical marker announced that it was one of Texaco's first.

The population seemed doubled the day we were there, too, what with all the people going up and down the streets and in and out of the shops. It was wonderful. We took a breather inside B & B Bygones for a special reason: they have an old-fashioned soda fountain at the back. My chauffeur had a plain coke float, but I zeroed in on a double chocolate soda, the likes of which I haven't had since I was a kid. Then we browsed through the shop, admiring all the antiques and collectibles in the cool, clean, air-conditioned shop.

Moving on, we drove to Gilmer along Highway 271 north, a nice, straight four-lane highway through the pines, with glimpses of the area's deep red earth at the edges. Sometimes vehicles turning onto the highway from unpaved roads left long red trails behind them on the pavement.

Turning west at Gilmer onto Highway 154, a Texas Forest Trail, we saw groups of cows huddled around hay mounds, busily munching. "I'd like to see how the machine that makes those mounds works," my companion said. "Replacing haystacks." The cows didn't seem to mind the change.

Highway 154, bordered alternately by stands of pines and fields of cattle, rolled up and down gentle hills. Just before Harmony the big pines made a lovely green canopy over the highway as we turned south on FM 312 to FM 49, which was hilly and curving, a regular roller-coaster ride in several parts. Then we entered Mineola.

Mineola is a town that takes its history seriously, especially its railroad history. The town developed in 1871 when the Great Northern Railroad was built through the area. Mineola was named by railroadman Ira H. Evans, and he named it after his daughter Ola, and her friend Minnie Patton. When you tell people this, they think it's a spoof, but no, it's historical fact. Known as the "Gateway to the East Texas Pine Country," Mineola is colorful a great deal of the year. The town sponsors wonderful trails through the wildflowers in the spring: dogwood, bluebonnets, and crimson clover, and in the fall the hardwood trees turn all shades of crimson, yellow, and gold among the evergreen pines.

We visited the Railroad Museum, housed in an old depot on Front Street, fronted by an old red caboose. We bought ourselves a pair of T-shirts with a big 'ol black engine roaring across the white front.

There's a great inn in town, the Munzesheimer Manor, a lovely restored 1898 mansion, in case you want to spend the night and be fed a fulsome breakfast.

Heading north on Highway 37, we looked forward to Quitman, which has quite a bit of history of its own. Since this was the hometown of James Stephen Hogg, first native-born governor of Texas, we weren't surprised to find Governor Hogg Shrine and State Park there. The family has been prominent in Texas history and politics, and we enjoyed both the Miss Ima Hogg Museum and the "Honeymoon Cottage" of her parents, James and Sarah Ann (Sallie) Hogg. In his early days, James Hogg published the *Quitman Daily News* (1873), later he was justice of the peace, then county attorney, and state attorney general. It was the road to the governorship evidently, an office which he held from 1891 to 1895.

It was time to leave Quitman, so we drove down Texas Forest Trail FM 2088 to FM 312 to Winnsboro, a town named after John E. Wynn, an early settler. Noticing the spelling, we had to ask, "What happened to the Y?" Seems like the spelling was changed in the 1870s by a newspaper editor who had a shortage of *y*s in his type. "You can't count on anything in this world," commented my philosophical companion.

Back in Civil War days Winnsboro was pretty pro-Confederate, and many of the mansions with their stately white columns reflect that antebellum feeling. Downtown there are several antique shops (though not near so many as in Gladewater!) and three churches. Winnsboro holds an Autumn Trails every weekend in October, and the bright foliage among the green pines is beautiful to see.

From Winnsboro we took FM 852 south, back to FM 2088 east, passing black-and-white and brown-and-white cattle munching on the hay mounds heaped on both sides of the road. We met up with FM 556 and turned toward Pittsburg. We weren't surprised to find a Pittsburg here, because Texas is supposed to have at least one place, however small, named after just about every other city in the world.

From Pittsburg we went east on FM 993 to FM 2254, where we startled two graceful deer on the quiet and deserted road. One bounded away immediately, but the other one took a few seconds to stop and boldly stare at us, the interlopers in this forest hideaway.

The road led us to Highway 297, past the huge edifices of Lone Star Steel and through the town of Lone Star to the road we were looking for, FM 729 east across the northern edge of Lake O' the Pines. The 18,700-acre lake was built by the U.S. Army Corps of Engineers as a reservoir amid the scenic rolling forest lands of East Texas. Fishing? Huge smallmouth buffalo weighing 97 pounds have been caught here, as have white bass weighing more than 12 pounds. On FM 729 we drove through heavily wooded land thick with solid pines, barely glimpsing the lake to our right until the road crossed over an arm of water jutting out. Then we could see how large and lovely the lake is; Lake O' the Pines is considered one of the most attractive lakes in East Texas, and we enjoyed driving alongside it, watching it glisten through the pines.

Three more miles of FM 729 and we coasted into Jefferson.

Jefferson, on Big Cypress Bayou, is a small town that has made tourism a big business, and there are more bed-and-breakfast inns here than you can count. More than 30 structures bear state historical medallions. Nobody's certain of the date the town began; various numbers between 1836 and 1840 are cited, but one thing is certain: as a major East Texas river port of entry, Jefferson was a thriving city in the 1870s. Big Cypress was navigable back then, and steamboats came streaming in from New Orleans on the Mississippi, into the bayou by way of nearby Caddo Lake.

However, the railroads, they were a-coming. But Jefferson, confident of the steamboat trade, refused to let railroad magnate Jay Gould mess up the town with his noisy engines. They said they'd rather have grass grow in the streets than his tracks, and furious, Gould predicted the death of the town. Die it did, until tourism and interest in Texas history revived it.

So we were intrigued. We had to visit the great Gould's private railroad car, the "Atalanta," permanently grounded on West Austin Street. The car has four staterooms, a lounge, dining room, kitchen, butler's pantry, and bathroom, and is delightfully 1890s ornate.

The Jefferson Historical Museum has four rather musty floors of documents, antiques, and other mementos of the past. More refreshing were visits to several of the town's beautifully restored mansions: the Captain's Castle, the Culberson House, Freeman Plantation, House of the Seasons, and Roseville Manor. The Captain's Castle is also a bed-and-breakfast inn run by a delightful retired couple.

Not only does Jefferson have history, several of its chefs are making culinary history. Stillwater Inn (a bed-and-breakfast inn) boasts another great chef-owner who offers such entrées as grilled breast of duck served with potatoes pureed with garlic and cream, a carrot terrine, and herbed zucchini.

Dessert? I tried Concord cake, a rich confection of chocolate mousse, meringue, whipped cream, and almonds.

Next on our route was Caddo Lake, and to get there we drove south on Highway 59 to FM 2208 east. There the road curved through the trees, opening up now and then to wide green vistas, until we reached FM 134 and turned south toward the lake. Cattle were still grazing the fields, and we passed a lovely white-columned mansion set far back on our left. "I wonder what its doing there," said my companion. "Do you realize that in 22 miles we've passed only two cars?" This is one of the nicest aspects of these lovely Texas Forest Trails—the lack of traffic. Almost without exception, we had the roads to ourselves, especially on the farm-to-market (FM) roads.

Lee's Grocery marked the corner where FM 134 turned into Highway 43 and we crossed over Highway 43 to continue on FM 2198 to Caddo Lake State Park. The park occupies 480 lovely wooded acres beside Caddo Lake on land once occupied by Caddo Indians, a tribe advanced in what is considered civilization. To learn something about them, we visited the park's interpretive center. Next we explored a small part of the nature trails before retracing the two miles back to Highway 43. Driving west along this Texas Forest Trail a short way, we reached Karnack, set back off the highway. (There's a sign.)

Karnack may be named for Karnak, Egypt, but it's renowned as the birthplace of Lady Bird Johnson. She was born Claudia Taylor, daughter of prosperous merchant T. J. Taylor. The town's not much more than a stop in the road, but it has an eating place, the Karnak Café, which advertises TRUCKERS WELCOME on a big wooden board out front. We couldn't imagine what truckers would come—until we learned that Thikol Chemical Corporation here makes the fuel that sends our rockets roaring into space! It wasn't until then that we noticed the huge storage tanks set off the road in the shrubbery. Across from the café we saw a church, and from the expression on the face of the gentleman waiting outside the church door, on Sunday he expected us to be in there, not looking for eats in the café. The café cooperated with a sign in the window saying CLOSED WEEKENDS.

Lady Bird's actual birthplace is down the road a piece, set well back behind an expanse of green lawn on the corner of Highway 43 and FM 2682. It's a handsome two-story building on a sloping hill, constructed of bricks made by slaves. The marker in front says Harrison County Historical Site, but it's not open to the public, so we drove on to Marshall.

Marshall, settled in 1839, was one of the largest and wealthiest cities in the state when Texas seceded from the Union in 1861. It began to produce saddles, harnesses, clothing, gunpowder, and ammunition for the Confederacy. When Vicksburg fell, Marshall became the seat of civil authority west of the Mississippi. We admired the Confederate Monument on the courthouse lawn; as for the building itself, it's a youngster, built in 1966, a tan-yellow beauty with white trim and a big white dome on top. It's no longer used as a courthouse, however; it houses the Harrison County Historical Society Museum.

The museum has interesting exhibits of Caddo Indian artifacts as well as pioneer and Civil War displays. For a change from history, we visited Frank's Doll Museum and gawked at some 1,600 dolls, doll furniture, and toys in yet another of Marshall's historic homes. We were lucky to catch Frank, because this museum is mainly open by appointment.

The Ginocchio National Historic District, three square blocks in the heart of the old downtown area, centers around the old Ginocchio Hotel, a Victorian masterpiece of an old railroad hotel. We had to admire it from the outside because it's "open occasionally." The streets leading to the hotel are lined with historic homes, and Marshall has more than half a dozen bed and breakfast places to stay.

Marshall Pottery is one of the area's oldest pottery factories still in operation; it's the largest manufacturer of red clay pots in America—all that red earth we passed throughout East Texas! We watched potters turn lumps of the native Texas clay into beautiful and functional pieces and then browsed through the 100,000 square feet of pottery and gifts for sale.

Leaving Marshall, we headed west on I-20 back to Longview.

For More Information

Gladewater Chamber of Commerce, (903) 845-5501 or (800) 627-0315

Mineola Chamber of Commerce, (903) 569-2087

Munzesheimer Manor (Mineola), (903) 569-6634

Quitman Chamber of Commerce, (903) 763-4411

Governor Hogg Shrine, (903) 763-2701

Thee Hubbell House (Winnsboro), (903) 342-5629

Marion County Chamber of Commerce (Jefferson), (903) 665-2672

The Captain's Castle (Jefferson), (903) 665-2330

Stillwater Inn (Jefferson), (903) 665-8415

Caddo Lake State Park, (903) 679-3351

Marshall Chamber of Commerce, (903) 935-7868

Frank's Doll Museum (Marshall), (903) 935-3065

Marshall Pottery, (903) 938-9201

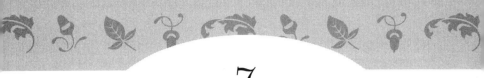

7

Cows, Ice Cream, and the Republic

Getting there: From Houston take State 249 north to FM 1774 to State 105 to Navasota. This trip covers sites related to two important events in Texas history: the founding of the Republic of Texas and the founding of Bell Ice Cream. We end in Austin, but you can also return to Houston on U.S. 290 east.

Highlights: Navasota and the La Salle Monument; Independence and the home of Sam Houston; Washington-on-the-Brazos and the Star of the Republic Museum; historic Chappell Hill; bluebonnets and Blue Bell Ice Cream in Brenham; Dime Box and Little Dime Box; Lexington; Elgin, home of the famous sausage; Manor, with Manor Downs.

We took State 249 north through Magnolia to FM 1774 and Plantersville. In season, in Plantersville, you can pick your own fruit in the King's Orchard (March to September). Strawberries, blackberries, raspberries, and blueberries grow there, as well as large juicy peaches, plums, and apples. (I ate more raspberries, my favorite fruit, than I picked to take along in the car. They were so delicious, right off the bush.)

When picking season is over, it's still not dull in Plantersville, because for seven weekends in October and November, the tiny town is the site of the Texas Renaissance Festival. There's medieval jousting, jesters, and minstrels—all in the name of fun, and the most fun is had by those who come in costume. Everyone goes around gnawing on huge turkey drumsticks. It was at the festival that I first came across that contradiction in terms, fried ice cream!

But we were between festival times, so we drove on to Navasota, changing to State 150 at Stoneham.

Navasota was a settlement as early as 1822, but it wasn't until 1859, when the Houston & Texas Central Railroad came to town, that it became an important shipping point—just in time for the Civil War.

What piqued our interest most was the monument to Robert Cavelier, Sieur de la Salle, who got himself and his men lost here while searching for the mouth of the Mississippi. He was way off base—his fleet of three ships wandered into Matagorda Bay around 1687. Still, undaunted, he established a coastal community called Fort Saint Louis. But instead of staying safely put, the trader-explorer wandered inland and was murdered, some say by Indians, others by one of his own men. In any event, he certainly looks handsome and imposing, standing 14 feet high on his monument on the grassy esplanade dividing State 90 downtown.

Navasota has a museum and several lovely Victorian homes. One of them, the LaSalle House, built in 1897, is a lovely Queen Anne Victorian, with a collection of antiques, collectibles, and both rare and antique books. It's at 412 E. Washington, and there are tours every Saturday and Sunday.

Next we followed State 150 south to FM 1155 into Washington, known historically as Washington-on-the-Brazos. This was the site in 1836 of the signing of the Texas Declaration of

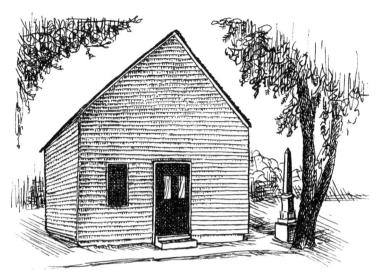

Washington-on-the-Brazos

Independence and the drafting of the Constitution of the newly born Republic of Texas. While it was busy becoming a flourishing retail and commercial center for the cotton grown in the Brazos River Valley, it even served briefly as the capital of the Republic, from 1842 to 1846 to be exact.

Washington-on-the-Brazos State Historical Park gave us a lot to look at, beginning with the Star of the Republic Museum. The star-shaped building is a repository of the history of the Republic, including the social life, agriculture, transportation, politics, and military affairs, all very attractively displayed.

The park itself contains part of the original town site, with a reconstruction of Independence Hall, a rustic log cabin, and in contrast, the elegant Barrington, home of the last President of Texas, Anson Jones. In between the two we found a shady pecan grove and partook of a pleasant picnic enjoying the shade and the breeze.

Next we followed in the footsteps of early settlers on FM 1155 through the beautiful pastoral landscape of the Brazos River Valley, to Chappell Hill.

Chappell Hill may have dwindled to a mere 310 folks today, but it was pretty important in its time. Settled in 1848, it soon had an institution of higher learning in the form of the Chappell Hill Female College. Today the small village has a historical museum and a local library, established in 1893, a self-service one to which the local inhabitants help themselves with their own keys!

Then it was time to turn west on U.S. 290 to Brenham, dairy country, famous for Blue Bell Creameries. Called locally "that little creamery in Brenham" when it was founded in 1907, officially it was the Brenham Creamery Company. The name was changed in 1930 in favor of the wildflower that grows profusely in the region, and ice-cream production rose from the 1911 output of two gallons a day to today's 20 million gallons a year.

That "little creamery" produces what a lot of people, including a national magazine, claim is the best ice cream in the entire country. Blue Bell invented such innovative flavors as cookies-and-cream, and others have jumped on that bandwagon. Naturally, we wanted to taste the delicious treat at the source, so we joined a free tour that ended with plenty of free sampling! (There are no tours on Saturday or Sunday, the plant is closed then.)

The county seat of Washington County, Brenham was settled on part of a league of land granted under the colonization laws of Coahuila (Mexico) and Texas. The town's strong German flavor was supplied by the many German immigrants who arrived in the 1860s, along the present-day Texas Pioneer Trail, which covers a four-county area. The Washington County Chamber of Commerce has a map.

In the spring, Brenham is famous for its Bluebonnet Trails, when the fields are blanketed with this pretty Texas State Flower. Of course there are poppies and primroses too, and

Indian paintbrush and a host of others, making Brenham a flower wonderland.

That's only in spring, of course, but Ellison's Greenhouses produces a year-round crop of foliage, mums, African violets, and such (you can visit on Fridays and Saturdays).

In Brenham's Firemen's Park, we spotted a wonderful sight, a beautiful carousel just waiting for passengers. What a disappointment to learn that only group tours can hitch a ride, and then only by reservation! But the vintage merry-go-round with Hershell-Spillman antique animals was a pleasure to look at all the same. "It's one of only 12 in Texas," we were told.

There are several historic homes worth looking at in Brenham, especially the Ross-Carroll-Bennett House and the Steinbach House. We loved the latter's gingerbread trim, not only along the porches, but under the eaves and up the gable.

Leaving Brenham, we started north on FM 50 toward Independence, but detoured to the right onto State 105 to visit the St. Clare Monastery Miniature Horse Farm.

The cloistered order of nuns built their present home in Brenham in 1986, and today their horses bring approximately $1,500 for a good quality pet, $5,000 for a show and breeding horse, and up to $15,000–$20,000 for a champion. Evidently this is big business: Monastery St. Clare horses are entered in 15 shows a year, including the Houston Stock Show, where 150–200 horses from all over the country compete.

Everyone who sets eyes on miniature horses is immediately captivated by these little charmers. Why not take one home for a pet? It's certainly not impossible and even not too impractical: they eat very little and require very little space. "A good size backyard will hold a pair of them," trainer John Garza told us. "They don't smell, they're not noisy, and they won't disturb the neighbors. They require only a handful of feed a day and the grass in the yard."

A miniature horse is an exact replica of a standard horse—except for its size. An average height of 27 inches is considered ideal, although some are as tall as 33 inches.

"You want to imagine that you're looking at an Arabian or a quarter horse or a draft horse, only small," Garza said. Well, it was tempting, but . . .

Instead, we turned back to FM 50 and drove north to Independence to see the Sam Houston Homesite. Houston was a giant among Texas historical figures, and we went prepared to be impressed. The village (pop. 140) was settled in 1824 by the family of John P. Coles, one of Stephen F. Austin's original three hundred families in Texas. At first it was called Cole's Settlement, but in 1836 it was changed to commemorate Texas's independence from Mexico. Next, the town square was laid out to accommodate a Washington County courthouse, but the settlement was doomed to disappointment: Brenham won the honor by a heated county-seat election, winning by all of two votes!

Independence today is just a crossroads, of FM 50 and FM 390. The Sam Houston Homesite on 390 is marked with a large granite marker, across from the entrance to the old Baylor University campus. We were surprised to learn that Independence was not only the birthplace of Waco's Baylor University but of Belton's Mary Hardin-Baylor College as well. All that's left of the original administration and classroom building are four large stone pillars. We didn't go look for more ruins on the six-acre original campus.

The Texas Baptist Historical Center on the crossroads consists of a museum and a church organized in 1839. Sam Houston was baptized here in 1854, which made his wife, Margaret Lea, mighty pleased. (The story goes that he'd been baptized Catholic when that's what was needed to get that all-important permission from Mexico to allow him to begin colonization in Texas of Anglos from the States and Europe.)

From Independence we took FM 390, following scenic curves through rolling country dotted with green trees, through Burton to FM 1697, where we began to see pump

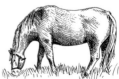

jacks working away in the flat green pastureland. The horses and cattle simply ignored them, going on about their business of grazing.

The road led us to FM 141 and into Dime Box, which we'd always been curious about. I mean, every visitor wants to know the origin of the name, and we were no exception. Evidently back in the "good old days" the custom was to put a dime in your mailbox for mail delivery. We found a marker to the custom on FM 141 at the corner of Slayton Avenue. It's a short rock pedestal topped by a glass case containing a huge silver dime. What made Dime Box more famous than its name was the visit in 1946 of President Franklin Delano Roosevelt, accompanied by NBC, to open the first March of Dimes office, right here in Dime Box.

Leaving Dime Box, we drove on through Little Dime Box (we didn't see anything worth stopping for) and on to Lexington via State 21 north for a few miles and then west on FM 696.

Lexington is the oldest settlement in its county, Lee, and it dates from the early 1850s. As in so many small villages, the arrival of the railroad put the town on the map. The business and population growth has not continued; Lexington is home to less than a thousand. But they are very friendly folks.

We stopped at the Lexington Mercantile Company and were greeted by Rebecca Green, third-generation proprietor of the old-fashioned store. Her mother, Charlotte Hooper, often bakes the goodies displayed in a glass case at the back of the store, and when she doesn't, Rebecca fills in. We tried one of each of the six homemade cookie flavors. (We split them in half; they're pretty good size!)

I fell for the chocolate chip, but my companion liked the peanut butter cookie best. That's fitting, because Lexington is big peanut-growing country. There used to be a festival in honor of it, the Gooberama. It was dropped, we were told sadly down at City Hall, because there wasn't enough interest in it.

Mercantile helper Nell Poston's husband Jerry is busy building an exact to-scale replica of Lexington from the 1940s, and we were invited then and there to drive down and take a look at it. It was amazing, an entire town laid out on a table in a small building back of the house. Jerry said he'd be happy to have people stop by and take a look at his creation any time; stop in the store and ask for directions.

From Lexington we turned back onto FM 696 west down to Elgin, which is famous for its hot sausage. Driving down the Main Street Historical District, we stopped at the Elgin Pharmacy, having heard rumors of an old-fashioned soda fountain there. We were doomed to disappointment. "It's long gone," they told us. So we went to find the old Elgin Sausage Company's restaurant on the railroad tracks, and *it* was gone, too—moved to the outskirts of town!

The only thing left for us was to drive west on U.S. 290 to Manor, where we had a satisfactory down-home meal at Cafe 290, which has been feeding home cooking to country folk since 1948.

The buffet special of chicken enchiladas, beans, and rice was hearty and filling, and there were carrots and boiled cabbage for extras if we needed our veggies.

Manor is home of Manor Downs, and there's racing on Saturdays and Sundays in the fall.

We headed into Austin on U.S. 290 west, passing the Austin Flea Market on the right five miles outside town. (If you want to return to Houston, just turn around on 290 and drive the 156 miles back.)

For More Information

King's Orchard (Plantersville), (409) 894-2766

Grimes County Chamber of Commerce (Navasota), (409) 825-6600 or (800) 252-6642

Washington County Chamber of Commerce (Brenham), (409) 836-3695

Washington-on-the-Brazos State Historical Park, (409) 878-2214

Blue Bell Creameries (Brenham) (call for tour hours), (800) 327-8135

The Monastery of St. Clare (Brenham), (409) 836-9652

Lexington Chamber of Commerce, (409) 773-4337

Lexington Mercantile Company, (409) 773-2231

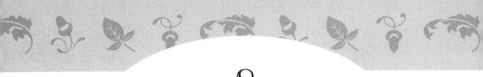

8

Seashore and the Big Thicket

Getting there: From Houston: take I-45 south to Galveston to State 87 along the coast. This trip explores the Texas coast east of Houston and heads north into Big Thicket country, returning via State 146 and U.S. 90 to Houston.

Highlights: The Bolivar Ferry; seashore and seafood along the Bolivar Peninsula; the Big Thicket National Preserve on Texas's southeast border; the Alabama-Coushatta Indian Reservation; Liberty, one of the oldest settled areas of Texas and home to Sam Houston's law practice.

Driving the 50 miles to Galveston through the flat countryside along I-45 made us eager to reach the high causeway arching over Galveston Bay onto Galveston Island. That's always the signal that the good part of the drive is going to begin.

Galveston, with its many beaches, museums, and parks, is a full-scale adventure alone, so saving it for another day, we swooped down off the causeway as I-45 became Broadway. The esplanade, aflame with pink blooming oleanders, made us remember that we were in a semitropical climate.

We turned right at 53rd Street, which led to the water, so we could enjoy the sea wall as we drove east toward U.S. 87

and the Bolivar Ferry. The sea wall was built after the hurricane of 1900 practically wiped Galveston out. We could see the high-water marks still clear on some of the old buildings that survived.

The Texas Highway Department operates several toll-free ferries in the state, and this one is a favorite for tourists and locals alike—as well as for overgrown children like my husband and me. Every 20 minutes one of these ferries leaves Galveston, and Port Bolivar on the other side, passing each other on the 15-minute boat ride across Galveston Bay.

Sometimes there's quite a long line, and we were amused to read the not-so-funny signs proclaiming: UNLAWFUL TO PASS VEHICLE FOR FERRY ACCESS and LINE CUTTING PROHIBITED— UP TO $200 FINE. You can be sure we stayed in line, and although we just missed an outgoing ferry, another one came along in just a few minutes. (But at other times we've had to wait quite a while. I could tell about one hot summer day, entertaining visiting Yankee cousins and their children . . .) Shining white, each ferry is trimmed in a different color—red, blue, green, or yellow.

After we'd followed the instructions to turn off our motor and set the parking brake, we climbed out of the car and joined the crowd enjoying the cool salt breezes. As we sailed across the bay, seagulls wheeled overhead and we looked (in vain that day) for the dolphins who often come along to play. Fishing boats in the distance were trailed by large flocks of gulls, beating the air with their wings to stay in place while they looked for a lucky windfall.

The ferry empties onto State 87, which follows along the narrow strip of the Bolivar Peninsula dividing Galveston Bay from the Gulf of Mexico, and all along the way we saw beach houses on both sides, built up on tall stilts in case hurricane tides and other high water comes raging up on the shores. (The space makes a great parking spot for the owner's cars.) We caught glimpses of shining water on both sides as we drove along the narrow peninsula.

At first we passed a lot of shell shops and seafood restaurants; then we began to notice pump jacks working away as we neared High Island, and we wondered whether there was much offshore drilling nearby, since there seemed to be oil here. Far off in the distance in the Gulf of Mexico, we could see big freighters and tankers.

At High Island we turned north on State 124 to aim for the Big Thicket. We drove high over another causeway, this time over the Gulf Intracoastal Waterway, and toward the small settlements of Stowell and Winnie south of I-20. Noticing all the marshes leading to beaches, I wondered aloud whether there were any alligators in the vicinity. "You bet," said my traveling companion. "Raccoons, too." Which is not quite the same thing!

Turning off 124 left onto FM 65 into Winnie, we stopped up the road a piece at Al-T's Seafood and Steakhouse, right on our route. Since Al-T's also specializes in Cajun food (being less than an hour's drive from the Louisiana border), we feasted on delicious gumbo, red beans and rice, and homemade cornbread.

Back in the car, we continued north, crossing I-10 onto FM 1663. We drove along field after field of sorghum, past huge groups of silver silos bunched together in the midst of open fields, before turning west on FM 365 through Nome. Just beyond Nome a roadside stand advertised "Fresh okra for sale."

Wide green fields became punctuated with slender lines of trees on the horizon. The land was as flat as a tortilla, with more pump jacks bobbing here and there. Then the road crossed U.S. 90, and from there we took FM 326 through Sour Lake and crossed over Little Pine Island Bayou. The stands of trees began to thicken, and we realized we were heading into Big Thicket country as we neared Kountze.

The town is surrounded by the Big Thicket; in an area that is more than 89 percent forested, Kountze calls itself "The Big Light in the Big Thicket." It was established as a railroad town in 1881, and today produces more than 5.5 million board feet of lumber annually.

Outside of Kountze, mention the Big Thicket and someone is sure to say "I've heard of it, but—what is it?" That's a fair question, because this vast tangle of often impenetrable woods, streams, and marshes, defined by the dictionary as a concentration of trees and shrubs, is, to the layman, a mysterious, vague, bewildering place.

But the Big Thicket is much more than that. Comprised of an entire 50-square-mile section of southeast Texas, bounded on the north by U.S. 190, on the east by the Neches River, on the south by U.S. 90, and the west by the Trinity River (a mere 85,500 acres is the national preserve), to a scientist it's an area of immense plant and animal diversity, produced by complex interactions between soil formations, climate, and drainage. The result is a variety of unusual plant associations, from arid pine sandylands to wet baygulls (low wet areas that originally were river channels) to floodplains.

We checked with the Big Thicket Information Station on FM 420, seven miles north of Kountze, before we took a short walk on one of the trails. We found fanlike palmettos, normally found in the Florida Everglades, growing next to reindeer moss from the Arctic! Rare and endangered plants are at home here, and the contrast is amazing: orchids and carnivorous plants flourished alongside common ferns.

Although we didn't see any, an incredible variety of animal life is at home in the thicket. Armadillos, bobcats, grey fox, squirrels, rabbits, and woodchucks evidently know their way around the maze. Birders find hummingbirds, herons, egrets, roadrunners, and all sorts of unusual songbirds, but you'd have to hang around longer than we did. We weren't too eager to meet up with any 12-foot-long alligators, or any of the 22 species of snake, which includes several varieties of rattlers, although we could have handled the five species of turtle, from small musk ones to the snapping turtles we were told can weigh up to one hundred pounds.

After our short hike in the woods, we drove off toward Saratoga on FM 770 to visit the Big Thicket Museum. It displays backwoods memorabilia like pioneer tools, artifacts, and documents. Then we headed for Woodville at the northern edge of the Big Thicket via a rather indirect route because we wanted to stay on country roads. First we followed FM 787, which took us through tall pines to FM 2798, where the small town of Votaw skirts the edges of the thicket. We hit a bumpy stretch just before Segno and turned east on FM 943 to FM 1276. The road became more hilly and curving as we crossed Big Sandy Creek. It was a great get-away-from-it-all road; there was no traffic, and no towns for a long while, just quiet woodsy wilderness.

When we reached U.S. 190, a Texas Forest Trail, we turned east toward Woodville, crossing Big Sandy Creek again, as well as Bear Creek and Mill Creek. But we hadn't gone very far when we came to the Alabama-Coushatta Indian Reservation. Of course we drove in, especially after seeing the Native American design signs saying ON TI CHUKA, which is Alabama-Couchatta for "Welcome."

The Alabama-Couchatta Indians of East Texas have lived in this Piney Woods region of the Big Thicket for more than three hundred years. During the Texas War of Independence from Mexico they maintained total neutrality, determined to remain peaceful and free. Sam Houston, a staunch friend of these southern forest tribes, was influential in creating the reservation in 1850.

Since settling on the reservation in the 1850s, the Alabama-Couchatta have developed an entire village of attractions exhibiting their culture, craftsmanship, and history. The Village is an authentic re-creation organized in exactly the way the Indians lived in the past. Tribal members employing traditional skills weave baskets and make jewelry, pottery, and leather items.

We found intricate beadwork fashioned into ties, belts, and other accessories, and one-of-a-kind pieces crafted in the Pottery Works. (They're for sale in the gift shop.)

The Indian History Museum tells the tale of the myths, legends, and battles of the tribe, from its roots in Alabama to its migration and settlement here in East Texas. Tribal dances are performed, but we weren't fortunate to be visiting at the right time. It was time to head on into Woodville, another town in the forest, east on U.S. 190. But to get there we had to cross Big Sandy Creek again (how that creek wanders!) as well as Woods Creek and Horse Pen Creek.

Woodville was named for George T. Wood, second governor of Texas, and the name is apt, because Woodville is a commercial center for lumbering and forest products. The area is almost 90 percent forested, and that means a lot of trees. The Heritage Village Museum features old buildings, shops, and homes, as well as records of Woodville life from pioneer days up to the Roaring Twenties.

The courthouse on the square was built in the 1890s and was remodeled in 1936, which we decided was kind of too bad after seeing photos of the original building. It had a lot more charm then, but I guess you couldn't stop "progress" any better back then than you can now!

There's a pretty bed-and-breakfast place in town, the Antique Rose, with roses everywhere: in the yard, at the front door, and even on most of the wallpaper.

The beautiful restored Victorian home at 302 North Charlton Street houses the Shivers Library and Museum. It was bought by former Texas Governor Allan Shivers and his wife, who restored it and then donated it to the city. Carpeting from France is part of the handsome furnishings, and the building is stocked with mementos and documents pertaining to Shivers's administration.

After a cozy stay in friendly, small Woodville, we retraced our route on U.S. 190 to Livingston, another lumber community. We found the Polk County Museum, which had quite an eclectic assortment of exhibits, from Early American glassware to Indian artifacts to a 1700s candelabra from the White House! Interesting was the historic log cabin of pioneer Jonas Davis, conveniently relocated downtown.

From Livingston we drove south toward Houston on State 146, passing through Liberty, which is among the oldest settled areas of Texas. Sam Houston practiced law here, and the Sam Houston Regional Library & Research Center is a repository of history of the 10 counties originally carved from the Atascosito-Liberty district of the Republic of Mexico.

In case we weren't sure that Liberty meant business, we were convinced when we saw the replica of Philadelphia's original Liberty Bell in the Geraldine D. Humphreys Cultural Center.

Inspired by both Texas and American liberty, we turned southeast onto U.S. 90 and headed back to Houston.

For More Information

Al-T's Restaurant (Winnie), (409) 296-9818

Tyler County (Woodville) Chamber of Commerce, (409) 283-2632

The Antique Rose (Woodville), (409) 283-8926

Livingston Chamber of Commerce, (409) 327-4929

Liberty-Dayton Area Chamber of Commerce, (409) 336-5736

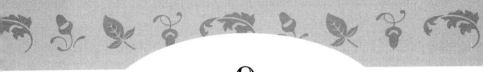

9

Up in the Panhandle to Canyon Country

Getting there: From Amarillo take State 136 north to Fritch on Lake Meredith, then make a circle east to Pampa, south on State 70, west on State 256, and north on State 207, returning to Amarillo on I-40 via U.S. 287. (It's a good idea to carry water when you drive in West Texas, both for drinking, and for the radiator—just in case.)

Highlights: Alibates National Monument and Lake Meredith; site of the Battle of the Adobe Walls at Stinnett; tanks and towers of oil and petrochemicals in now-tame Borger; White Deer Museum in Pampa; the spectacular scenery of Palo Duro Canyon, historic Tule Canyon (at the edge of Cap Rock from Brice to Silverton), and north to Claude.

From Amarillo we took State 136 north toward Fritch, past flat farmland. "Forage crops. Sorghum." announced my knowledgeable husband, for all the world like a farmer. Is all Texas covered with sorghum? We sure have seen a lot. That he didn't know.

On the left a copper refinery stood out in the wide open country. "Look," he said suddenly, pointing to the right. There was a rancher, driving his pickup right onto the field. Immediately all the cattle that had been spread out over the fields pushed and shoved themselves closely around the truck, just like a flock of sheep. "Guess he came to feed them, and they must be well trained!" As we drove on, we noticed more cattle, clustered around watering holes on both sides of the highway, reminding us that we were in pretty dry country. The barbed-wire fences on both sides of the road reminded us that we were in cattle country, and the occasional pump jack, that we were in oil country. Drought, cattle, and oil—that's the Texas Panhandle.

After a while we passed Lake Meredith and the Alibates National Monument. The lake, we knew, had been made by damming the Canadian River. Curious about the monument, we stopped and discovered that the site was the Alibates Flint Quarries, administered by the National Park Service. Here for thousands of years people have been quarrying flint; in fact, archaeological traces of prehistoric Indians—their homes, workshops, and campsites—dot the entire Canadian River region of the Texas Panhandle.

For 12,000 years people quarried flint for toolmaking. Indians of the Ice Age Clovis Culture used Alibates flint for spear points when they went to hunt the Imperial mammoth. It was awesome to learn that this occurred even before the Great Lakes were formed.

"The flint usually lies just below the surface at ridge level, in layers up to six feet," the park ranger told us. (Admission to the park is by tour only, so if you don't get there between Memorial Day and Labor Day, you have to contact the superintendent, since off-season tours are given by reservation only.)

Flint was gathered and used by nomadic peoples for most of the quarry's history. Between A.D. 1150 and 1500 farming

Indians who lived in the area grew corn, beans, and squash, using the drylands method of placing plants far apart to capture whatever sparse soil moisture they could. But they also quarried flint to use as tools in hunting bison, antelope, deer, and turkey, and for trade as well.

Ancestors of the Plains Village Indians such as the Pawnee or Wichita Indians, these early peoples were driven out of the area by aggressive Indians from the west. By the end of the 15th century, along came nomadic tribal hunters like the Apaches, Comanche, and Kiowas, introducing the Plains stage, from 1500 to 1875.

They had their day, too, until horses and European trade goods were introduced and eventually Anglo military campaigns and eastern buffalo hunters ended the Indian occupation. (And almost succeeded in finishing off the buffalo as well!)

Capturing some of the flint, or any of the rocks on the site, for your own collection is prohibited at Alibates, so we were careful to keep our hands in our pockets.

Bemused by thoughts of so long ago, we drove into Fritch, a friendly, small Panhandle town. In case we were in any doubt about its friendliness, we were greeted by a huge sign that proclaimed: HOWDY, NEIGHBOR, WELCOME TO FRITCH and was decorated with a happy face, the Lone Star flag, and the Texas state emblem.

Fritch has quite a remarkable aquarium and wildlife museum, a joint effort of the community and the National Park Service at Lake Meredith. Dioramas painted by local artist La Nelle Poling, who also has work in a museum in nearby Panhandle, are of actual locations in the area. They serve as backgrounds for the realistically mounted coyotes, turkeys, bobcats, raccoons, antelope, and other wildlife of the Panhandle.

The dioramas curve around the museum's main room, and down a few steps into the adjoining room, where large aquarium tanks exhibit the species of fish to be found in Lake Meredith. Walleye, largemouth and smallmouth bass, crappie, bluegill, perch, channel cat, yellow flathead catfish, and carp are all busily swimming around in the water.

One of the most important events in the history of Fritch was the building of the Sanford Dam and the construction of Lake Meredith on the Canadian River, just northeast of Fritch. Finished in 1965, the lake filled so rapidly that the builders had to work hard in a hurry to get the dam high enough to contain the water.

Lake Meredith lies on the dry and windswept High Plains of the Texas Panhandle, called the Llano Estacado, Spanish for Staked Plain. It's as flat as any surface in the world. Over eons of time the Canadian River cut and recut two-hundred-foot canyons called breaks, and the lake now fills those breaks. The long, narrow lake offers the usual pleasures of water sports such as boating, fishing, waterskiing, and sailing. Swimming, however, is at your own risk, and scuba diving is not recommended because of poor visibility.

From Fritch we took the scenic drive east on FM 136 over to FM 687 north through Sanford, joining FM 1319 there across the dam impounding Lake Meredith, and back on FM 687 north to Stinnett. The road crosses the rough canyon-cut landscape of the Canadian River breaks. We were eager to see the site of the Battle of the Adobe Walls, where two famous Indian battles were fought. One of them was Kit Carson's last fight.

We found that the site is some 18 miles northeast on private ranchland—not too accessible. But local directions were available, and we found historical markers there. What happened was this: in 1864 Carson and his U.S. troops narrowly escaped defeat by Kiowa and Comanche Indians, who had been molesting wagons trains and settlers. Then 10 years later, in 1874, near the site of the first battle, Indians under Quanah Parker and Lone Wolf attacked a stockade containing 28 men, buffalo hunters, and one woman. They attacked at dawn, and although they were repulsed, they surrounded the place, and it seemed only a matter of time before they would win the day.

But on the second day, a group of Cheyenne Indians appeared on the high mesa overlooking the camp, which set the stage for what has turned out to be a shot written down in history. From within the stockade, William (Billy) Boyd picked off an Indian on his horse at an unbelievable distance of almost seven-eighths of a mile. The story goes that the Indians were so shocked by this show of the white man's shooting ability that after mounting several desultory attacks, they withdrew.

From Stinnett, State 207 took us south down to Borger, at one time a wild oil boomtown.

Borger came into existence in 1926 following the discovery of the rich Panhandle Oil Field. A boomtown of tents and shacks sprang up, swelling the population to about 40,000. (Today it's about 15,500.) But order soon was applied, and Borger has grown into a center for oil, chemicals, and cattle, with tanks and towers of oil and petrochemical plants dominating the skyline.

The Hutchinson County Historical Museum displays exhibits from the time of Coronado's explorations to the boomtown days of the more recent past.

From Borger we took State 152 east to Pampa, past road signs for the small communities of White Deer and Goodnight, and past gathering tanks as well as more pump jacks and cattle. Pampa is named for *pampas*, the Spanish word for plains. A city of almost 20,000, it was founded in 1888 along the Santa Fe Railroad and today is an oil field supply point as well as market center for agriculture and livestock. Fourteen municipal parks on tree-shaded grounds give the city a spacious and verdant air unusual in the arid plains country.

"Being surrounded by lakes doesn't hurt, either," said my traveling companion. He'd noticed that no less than three lakes—Greenbelt, McClellan, and Meredith—surround the area.

The White Deer Land Museum in town has a mixed bag of exhibits. Records and documents of White Deer Land Company, established in 1882, are there, along with period rooms, a chapel, carriage house, and office, as well as exhibits depicting early ranching days with rooms containing furniture such as sideboards full of glass and china and cradles with original baby linen.

From Pampa State 70 led us south across I-40 and down to Clarendon, more flat land and pump jacks. As we drove south, the canyon country seemed to begin, but then it flattened out as we drove by irrigated crops of sorghum. Clarendon was established in 1878 by a Methodist minister as a "sobriety center"—as opposed to the wild Borgers and Pampas of the oil boom times. Local cowboys began to call it the "Saint's Roost," and we went to visit the Saints Roost Museum, housed in the former Adair Hospital. Cornelia Adair founded the hospital in 1910 for local cowboys, and the museum features heirlooms from ranches, farms, and businesses of the area.

Clarendon is the oldest town still alive and well in the Texas Panhandle. Fossilized specimens from the Clarendon Age dating back 11 million years to the Early Pliocene Age can be found in many a museum. While farming and ranching are the primary activities of the community, locals like to describe Clarendon as "home of trailblazers, cattle barons, cowboys, preachers, teachers, sodbusters, merchants, craftsmen, artists, old bones and old fossils . . . and maybe a few saints!"

Leaving Clarendon and passing up Bliven's Pharmacy and Health Mart (selling "Texas T-shirts at a bargain"), we crossed U.S. 287 and drove south on FM 70 through tiny Brice to State 256. As 256 curved from south to west and crossed Prairie Dog Town Fork of the Red River, a dramatic change in the scenery marked the eastern edge of the Great Plains of the United States. The road spiraled up jagged escarpments and beautiful scenic vistas to the edge of the High Plains, which the local residents call Cap Rock.

Silverton was formed as the county seat of Briscoe County when the county was organized in 1892. A commercial center for the immense farming and ranching area that includes the spectacular scenery of Palo Duro Canyon, Tule Canyon, and the edge of Cap Rock, it's one of only two towns in the entire county.

The Old Jail Museum, built in 1892, is an old stone building, the oldest in the county. For entry, we visited the county attorney's office in order to see the jail office and the cells upstairs. It's on courthouse square, with a restored windmill nearby.

Nearby Lake Mackenzie lies amid 910 acres of Tule Canyon, with facilities for picnicking, camping, boating, and swimming. Waterskiing, too, and of course fishing, for record-breaking catches of walleye, largemouth and striped bass, and catfish.

From Silverton we went north on State 207 across Palo Duro Canyon to Claude for another spectacular drive, considered one of the most impressive in Texas. As we reached Tule Canyon, we saw wonderful varieties of rock strata and sheer-faced knife-edged buttes. Then the highway plunged into the scenic grandeur of Palo Duro Canyon, formed, surprisingly, by a rather insignificant stream, the Prairie Dog Fork of the Red River, which we had crossed on State 256 from Brice. But that little stream had carved a canyon that extends one

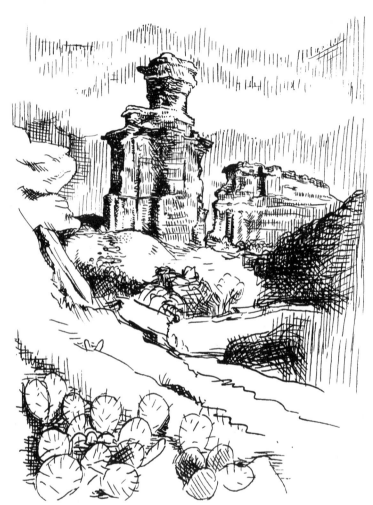

Palo Duro Canyon

hundred miles northwest to southeast and is nine miles wide, so it must have been much more than a little stream in pre-historic times!

We drove past a riot of colors—pink, orange, yellow, and green—on curves that took our breath away. We could see the road winding ahead of us until we reached the level land leading into Claude, where it changed suddenly to flat agricultural lands with more sorghum, and some cotton, stretching wide from one horizon to the other. Rather an anticlimactic end to all the splendor of the canyons behind us.

We found, no surprise, that Claude was born of the railroad. In 1887 it was established as a stop on the Fort Worth and Denver Railroad. Grain elevators and stockyards reveal the major agricultural production of today, although Claude is beginning to have a small reputation as an antique destination, due to the advent of several antique shops.

From Claude we took U.S. 287 west back to I-40 and returned to Amarillo.

For More Information

Amarillo Convention & Visitors Council, (806) 373-7800 or (806) 374-1497

Alibates National Monument and Lake Meredith Recreation Area, (806) 857-3151

Fritch Chamber of Commerce, (806) 857-2458

Borger Chamber of Commerce, (806) 274-2211

Pampa Chamber of Commerce, (806) 669-3241

Clarendon Chamber of Commerce, (806) 874-2421

10

Oil, Cattle, and Indians Along the Old Chisholm Trail

Getting there: From Abilene take I-20 east to Baird and on to State 6 north at Eastland. Then follow 6 north to Albany; continue on 6 to Stamford, then south on U.S. 277 to State 92 west through Hamlin to FM 57 south through McCauley, crossing I-20 at Sylvester to Sweetwater. Then State 70 south to FM 153 and over to Buffalo Gap via FM 126 and FM 89, ending on 89 back into Abilene.

Highlights: Baird, with two museums; Eastland, with "Old Rip," the horned frog; Albany and the Georgia Monument; Stamford and the Mackenzie Trail Monument; Sweetwater and buffalo hunters; Buffalo Gap and Buffalo Gap Historic Village; Fort Phantom Hill and Lake Fort Phantom Hill.

We left Abilene on I-20 east, going toward Baird, a city of a little more than 1,500 citizens that was established in 1880 with the building of the Texas and Pacific Railroad. "What Texas would have been like without the railroad, I hate to think," remarked my chauffeur-husband. In any event, the town was named for the official who drove the first stake into the ground in 1875, which seems to be his only claim to remembrance by posterity. The Railroad Heritage Museum & Library tells the whole tale in a 1911 depot, and the Callahan County Pioneer Museum tells tales of life on a pioneer farm and ranch.

From Baird we continued east on I-20 to Eastland, with twice as many citizens as Baird but only one museum, the Kendrick Religious Museum of biblical dioramas. Eastland's more unique claim to fame is "Old Rip," the horned frog.

Don't ask me why, but apparently a horned frog was sealed in a cornerstone of the original Eastland courthouse, built in 1897. Hard to believe, but when a new courthouse was built, the early cornerstone was opened and, lo and behold, there was a live horned frog! Displayed nationally, the small amphibian was quite a celebrity, and when it died the following year, it was placed in a glass-front casket and is on view in the courthouse to this day.

Another intriguing oddity of Eastland is the Post Office Mural, composed entirely of 12,000 postage stamps. It took seven years to stick all those stamps on the six-by-ten-foot mural.

At Eastland we left I-20 behind and drove north on State 6 to Albany, past industrious farmers digging holes for fenceposts. They were lagging behind their neighbors—both sides of the road on the surrounding flat farmlands beyond them were already fenced.

"Look at that dead possum on the road," my husband said suddenly, although he was going too fast for me to see it. I'd rather see a live one, anyway!

We drove to Albany through oil country, with both gathering tanks and pump jacks working away along the road. The land became gently rolling, with lots of green trees, and we passed a veritable mesquite forest on our right. Albany is a town of under two thousand but with a wingdinger of an annual celebration, the Fort Griffin Fandangle, presented by more than two hundred townsfolk under the West Texas starry skies of June. It's a musical version of Albany history as it's still remembered by the old-timers, a combination ballet and regular hoedown of laughter and tears

ALBANY, HOME OF THE HEREFORD is the sign that greeted us as we pulled into town. The seat of Shackelford County, Albany was an early supply point on the Western Trail to Dodge City. It's still important ranchland, since Albany's beef cattle account for 90 percent of the county's agricultural income. But we'd noticed all those pump jacks and gathering tanks and it was no surprise to learn that Albany is also an oil-producing and oil well supply center.

The town is proud of its newspaper, the *Albany News*, which was established in 1883 and has preserved valuable files of authentic frontier history, not only of its own past but also those of other frontier-era publications of the area.

Albany's famous Georgia Monument is not to the state of the same name, as you might expect. It was erected in 1976 to fulfill a longstanding promise to honor the Georgia Battalion that volunteered in the Texas War of Independence in 1836. Dr. John Shackelford, who was from Georgia, recruited 45 men to come to Texas in 1836 to fight the Mexicans.

When Mexican general Santa Anna massacred Colonel James Fannin's prisoners down in Goliad in savage violation of the honorary terms of surrender, many were from the Georgia Battalion.

Flags of the State of Georgia join the Lone Star of Texas and the U.S. flag as they fly over the stone marker and fountain. Plaques tell the story of the Georgians' contribution to the new Republic of Texas.

Dr. Shackelford, for whom the county is named, was spared only because the Mexicans thought he would be useful in treating wounded Mexican soldiers. He managed to escape, and although he returned to Georgia, Texas felt it owed him a lot. Hence the county name—and the monument.

Shackelford County Courthouse is a handsome structure, its exterior unchanged since it was built in 1883.

Fort Griffin was the supply base for the U.S. Army during its campaigns against the Comanches between 1872 and 1874. A few years later it served as a supply center for buffalo hunters when they moved into these southern plains. Some ruins still stand in Fort Griffin State Park off U.S. 283 north of town.

At the Old Jail Art Center we were amazed to discover works by such luminaries as John Marin, Charles Umlauf, Louise Nevelson, Modigliani, and Picasso, as well as Chinese art from the Ming, Han, Wei, T'ang, and Sui Dynasties. And all housed in a restored county jail from 1878!

There's also a restored frontier ranch house in Albany, complete with the rustic furnishings of the period. It's a typical dog-run cabin, with an opening in the center running from front to back so both sides of the house could catch a breeze. Instead of the more usual logs, the house is made of upright poles, or pickets.

We hated to leave Albany, but it was time to hit the road, since sticking to our itinerary meant continuing on State 6 west past the tiny towns of Lueders and Avoca. Except for crossing the Clear Fork of the Brazos River, the route was uneventful.

Another fork of the Brazos River, the South Fork, runs south into Fort Phantom Hill Lake just north of Abilene, but from where we were, there was no road to follow to the lake, so we decided to visit it after we returned to Abilene. We went on to discover Stamford's interesting sights.

Stamford is famous for its Texas Cowboy Reunion every year around the Fourth of July. It was started in 1930 and stands unchallenged as the greatest amateur rodeo in the world. Prizes include cash, trophies, and handmade saddles. Chuckwagons serve mouth-watering barbecue, and there's a major western art show.

Speaking of western art, Stamford's Texas Cowboy Museum has a collection of original paintings and prints by noted cowboy artists. The art is combined with farm and ranch artifacts from early in this century, including a living room/kitchen and a blacksmith shop.

The Mackenzie Trail Monument in Stamford is a large, hand-carved marker standing out under open skies. It was erected by descendants of early ranchers who wanted to represent what the famous Mackenzie Trail meant to area pioneers in the late 1880s. Carved into the stone are buffalo, cactus, Indians, cowboys, and oxen pulling a covered wagon, depicting frontier life in a nutshell. Only not a nutshell: the figures carved in the monument are almost life-size.

Leaving Stamford, we drove west across on State 92 to State 70, again crossing that Clear Fork of the Brazos as we headed south to Sweetwater, just barely north of I-20.

"It pays to advertise," said my driver, slowing down to read a highway sign that said MULBERRY MANSION. In town we learned that it was a beautiful bed-and-breakfast in a restored sanitorium, turned into a restful, luxurious place to spend the night.

Sweetwater began life as a store in a dugout that accommodated buffalo hunters in 1877. Today its 12,000 citizens have turned it into a banking and commercial center, with gypsum and cement plants, a cottonseed oil mill, and a garment manufacturer.

The Sweetwater Commercial Historic District is listed on the National Register of Historic Places; its buildings representing architectural styles spanning 40 years, from the 1900s through the 1930s.

The Pioneer City-County Museum has more than a dozen rooms displaying the lives of early settlers. If you want even more, there are extensive photographic files, as well as farm and ranch exhibits and Native American artifacts.

From Sweetwater we took the cutoff FM 1856 across I-20; it led to Lake Sweetwater. A spacious park surrounds the meandering 630-acre lake, and in addition to the usual fishing and water sports, there is also a golf course on the shore of the lake.

We followed 1856 around to where it ends at State 70 and turned south, enjoying the quiet country drive. When the road met up with FM 153, we turned east onto it toward Buffalo Gap. That took a little winding: we had to go south for about five miles and then east again on FM 126 through Nolan. When 126 turned north toward I-20, we took FM 89 on across Lake Abilene into Buffalo Gap.

Lake Abilene is another of Texas's many manmade lakes. It's accessible from both Abilene and Buffalo Gap, and folks enjoy the fishing, swimming, and boating here.

As for Buffalo Gap, it was a lot of fun. It got its name from its role as a natural pass through which buffalo traveled for centuries. In recent history it was a point on the famous Dodge Cattle Trail, and there are a lot of historic structures to visit at Buffalo Gap Historic Village.

In fact there are 20 buildings, a regular village set under live oak trees. All restored and furnished, they include a court-house/jail—rustic, of course, not your usual stone or brick town square centerpiece—a railroad depot, and a blacksmith and woodworking shop. Others are a 19th-century office of a doctor-dentist, a two-room schoolhouse, a bank from 1880, as well as buggies and wagons spread around, and exhibitions of firearms and Native American artifacts. We enjoyed all the old-time artifacts, including the kiddie horse ride, marked "10 cents," on the front porch of the general store.

We couldn't end our tour without taking a look at both Lake Fort Phantom Hill and Fort Phantom Hill. The lake, surrounded by paved highways that circle just about the entire 29 miles of shoreline, is south of the old fort ruins. Like most Texas frontier forts, Phantom Hill was established to protect the frontier from Indians. After suffering a series of hardships (mainly desertions) it was abandoned in 1854. Historians figure the desertions were due to monotony and loneliness. "Is it possible that the Indians didn't keep them busy enough?" my chauffeur wanted to know. In any event, the fort burned shortly after it was abandoned, leaving only chimneys and foundations as reminders. But the stone commissary, guardhouse, and powder magazine were spared, not being made of wood. We found interpretive signs telling us all about it.

Here's an amazing story about Abilene: Originally the city was a livestock shipping point on the Texas and Pacific Railroad, which made it a major cattle area. But in recent years oil has added to the city's economy, so when the city celebrated its centennial in 1981, an oil rig was set up in the county fairgrounds. It was intended just as a demonstration, to illustrate the technique of what oilmen call "making hole." By pure accident they struck oil. Not a lot, but enough to turn a modest profit! Can you believe such luck?

For More Information

Abilene Convention & Visitors Council, (915) 676-2556 or (800) 727-7704

Baird Chamber of Commerce, (915) 854-2003

Eastland Chamber of Commerce, (817) 629-2332

Albany Chamber of Commerce, (915) 762-2525

Stamford Chamber of Commerce, (915) 773-2411 or (800) 292-5635

Sweetwater Chamber of Commerce, (915) 235-5488

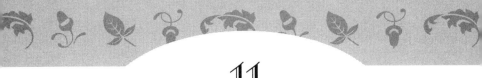

11

A Texas Lakes Trail

Getting there: From Fort Worth take State 199 across Lake Worth through Azle to FM 730 south, a Texas Lakes Trail, to Weatherford. Continue south on State 171 through Cresson to Cleburne. From Cleburne take U.S. 67 west to Glen Rose, then State 144 north to Granbury. From Granbury take FM 51/204 south to FM 2157 and west to Stephenville. Go north on U.S. 281 to FM 4, continue on FM 4 across I-20 to Palo Pinto. From there take U.S. 180 east to Mineral Wells and go north on U.S. 281, returning to Fort Worth on State 199.

Highlights: Eight lakes: Worth, Weatherford, Pat Cleburne, Squaw Creek, Granbury, Thorp Spring, Palo Pinto, and Mineral Wells; Weatherford, home of Mary Martin; Glen Rose, home of dinosaurs; Granbury, with pecans and the Nutt House; Mineral Wells and its Crazy Water Well.

Texas is dotted with lakes, all but one (Caddo Lake) manmade by damming the many rivers and river tributaries that wander all over the state. Heading west out of Fort Worth, the "Gateway to the West," we took State 199 across the broad waters of Lake Worth. The lake is known for its scenic vistas along Meandering Drive, which meanders indeed, all around most of the 3,560 acres of the lake. Turning south

89

at Azle, onto FM 730, we began our Texas Lakes Trail, narrow and winding through small hills. We passed signs cautioning us to be alert to deer, but we were disappointed not to see any. (They come out at night, and then you have to be careful not to hit one!) We crossed U.S. 180 and angled west into Weatherford on I-20.

We wanted to be in Weatherford for First Monday, held on the weekend preceding the first Monday of each month. The "trash and treasures" gathering evolved from trades day, when court was in session on the first Monday of the month, and farmers and ranchers took advantage of the crowds to bring produce and livestock to town. In addition to trash and treasures, we noticed there was still some livestock to be had for the bargaining!

Weatherford was the last settlement on the western frontier when wagon trains operated between Fort Worth and Fort Belknap. Weatherford's modern claim to fame is as the home of superstar Mary Martin. There's a statue of her in Peter Pan garb in front of the public library. Inside the library, there's a museum collection of works on the famous actress. Her childhood home, however, is not open to the public.

Oliver Loving's grave is in Weatherford. He was famous around these parts in the old days, known as "Dean of Texas Trail Drivers." He was wounded in 1867 by Indians, died, and was carried back to Weatherford to be buried. His son, along with driver Charles Goodnight, brought the body six hundred miles by wagon, and there's a historical marker over his grave.

In the southwest area of town, we found some gorgeous Victorian mansions built in the late 1800s. Two particularly grand ones, each on a high hill and claiming "the best view of the city" are bed-and-breakfasts: Victorian House and St. Botolph's.

If you have time for a walking, as well as a driving, tour of the city, the Chamber of Commerce in the old Santa Fe

Depot has maps. The depot itself is a restored 1909 brick structure, one of the first in the area to have a concrete floor. Leaving Weatherford, we backtracked a bit on I-20 to State 171, going south through Cresson to Cleburne. It was pretty green country, the road winding through small hills until it flattened out into ranch country. Around Cresson (pop. 208) there were some nice large ranch houses on both sides of the road. A huge banner hung over the road through Cresson, proclaiming CRESSON FALL FESTIVAL, but we weren't in time for that. We drove beside hayfields into Godley, where signs boasted 1988 LADY WILDCATS STATE CHAMPION BASKETBALL— pretty neat for a town with a population of 614!

We passed more sorghum fields and some goats, and then we were in Cleburne, with a population of more than 22,000. Mainly a commercial center of an agricultural area featuring dairy, livestock, and farming (which we could see as we drove by the fields and cattle), Cleburne surprised us by having Texas's largest railroad construction and repair shop industry.

"So many Texas small towns lived and died by the rails, it's a pleasant change to find one that's thriving from the 'iron monsters,'" remarked my companion. (Of course, they're not called that anymore.)

Cleburne's Leyland Museum contains fossils and Native American artifacts dating from pre-Columbian cultures as well as the more usual historic relics from the county (Johnson) and other early Texana.

Cleburne State Park, 12 miles southwest of town, contains a wildlife refuge as well as the usual swimming, boating, hiking, and camping facilities. Lake Pat Cleburne, named, as is the city, for Confederate General Pat Cleburne, is a 1,550-acre municipal lake owned by the city.

From Cleburne we headed west on U.S. 67 toward Glen Rose, along land fenced on both sides of the road and lined with large green cedars. We coasted down a hill and over a girder bridge on the Brazos River through Rainbow into Glen Rose, the dinosaur town. The road was hilly and a little bumpy, but the greens of municipal Squaw Valley Golf Course on our right were smooth as smooth.

Glen Rose is the home of Dinosaur Valley State Park on the Paluxy River. The river flows over solid rock, rock that contains the best-preserved dinosaur tracks in Texas, and the first sauropod tracks discovered in the world. The sauropods were plant-eating reptiles, more than 60 feet long and weighing 30 tons. The other tracks in the riverbed are those of the 30-foot-long duckbilled dinosaur and the 12-foot-tall meat-eating theropods.

Not all the tracks are covered with water, and it was quite a thrill to step where those dinosaurs had stepped one hundred million years ago! There are interpretive exhibits in the park, including a fenced-in area with two huge replicas of the prehistoric monsters. The 1,204-acre park also offers camping, picnicking, and nature trails.

The Somervell County Historical Museum is on courthouse square, along with Four Sisters Antiques, the Glen Rose Emporium, and Double T T-Shirts. The Inn on the River is housed in a renovated health sanatorium in case you want to spend the night and commune some more with the dinosaurs.

We took State 144 north to Granbury, another small town with big ideas, passing a cute little donkey standing wistfully behind a fence along the road. Other sights were a pretty picnic area on the right under big shade trees and a long white fence around the Happy Hill Farm (a children's home).

Granbury Square is on the National Register of Historic Places, and the county (Hood) is the largest producer of pecans in a state of pecans. (Texas's state tree is the pecan.) Particularly appropriate, then, is Granbury's Nutt House, even though the name is a coincidence, since the historic inn was built by the Nutt brothers, Jesse and Jacob, in 1893. Both bed and board were provided in the old days, and we enjoyed our

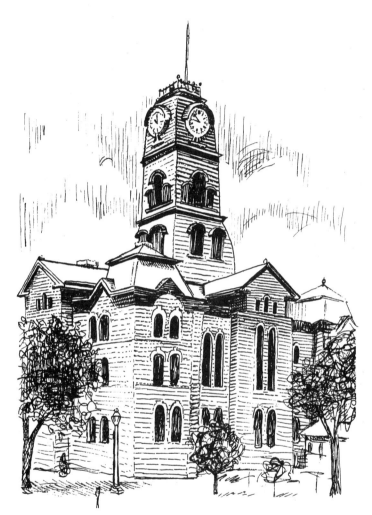

Hood County Courthouse

meal of chicken and dumplings and hot-water cornbread in the restaurant, just like in the old days.

The handsome Hood County Courthouse faces the Granbury Opera House, built in 1886. Restored in 1975 to its earlier glory, it presents musicals and plays to eager audiences on weekends February through December.

The Brazos River wanders all over this part of Texas, and Thorp Spring is an offshoot of it a little north of Granbury. But the town is right on Lake Granbury, and it edges the looping channel of the Brazos at the De Cordova Bend of the river. De Cordova Dam, which forms the 8,700-acre lake, was named for an early Texas entrepreneur, one Jacob de Cordova, who collected land scrip for a total of more than a million Texas acres. He billed himself as "Publicity Agent for an Empire," and in 1859 went a-lecturing back East to inspire interest in Texas.

It was time to go on to Stephenville, so we angled southwest on FM 51, past Glen Rose's Squaw Creek Lake to FM 204 and onto FM 2157 into Stephenville. Stephenville has one of the largest tree nurseries in the state, in case you're into reforestation. "It's tempting," my husband said. "We could use another tree in the backyard."

"Not in this car!" I protested. Instead, we went to see the Historical House Museum Complex, with its 1869 Victorian home furnished with period furniture and relics of the area's history. Stephenville is the seat of Erath County, named for Austrian George Erath. He fought at the historic Battle of San Jacinto (for Texas Independence) and served in the Texas Congress and later in the U.S. legislature. He surveyed this settlement in 1850 for the Stephens brothers. In fact, the original town site was donated by brother John M.—but frontier conditions made it rough in Stephenville until the 1870s, what with Indian attacks and all. Seems that just about all the men in town wore six-shooters, even the preacher, although it was reported that he laid his gun aside while preaching.

We didn't find any gun totin' in town, but that's not why we moved on. We wanted to continue our lake tour to Lake Palo Pinto and the town of the same name. We wandered north along State 108 through Huckabay to Thurber, a few miles west on I-20. We'd been surprised to learn of this coal mining town, which was founded in 1888 by the Texas & Pacific Coal Company (now owned by the Sun Oil Company). There isn't much left of Thurber, since the town was abandoned and almost entirely razed in 1933. A former company store building displays photographs of Thurber when its population grew to 10,000 with the discovery of coal. Miners were recruited from all over the world, and 17 nationalities were represented at one time. Next, high-grade clay was discovered, and brick manufacturing became a big industry. The mines closed in 1921 and the brick plant in 1930, but recent strip coal-mining might revive Thurber.

We retraced our route over I-20 and continued on to FM 4, which led past Lake Palo Pinto to Palo Pinto. We drove through Santo over gently rolling hills and lush greenery, along pecan orchards that made my companion's mouth water. In fact, he stopped to gather a few, but they weren't remotely ripe yet, to his disappointment.

Tiny Santo, like Godley on the way to Cleburne, had something to brag about. Emblazoned on the water tower were the words 1990 BASKETBALL CHAMP. Impressed, we drove on past open pastureland and cattle, and a surprise: a clump of prickly pear cactus, a type of vegetation we're more used to in the Hill Country and West Texas. But the ride was delightful. "Very pretty land in here," said my driver. "This is exactly what I think a country ride should be." He was remembering some of our West Texas drives, where we didn't see much besides flat open land.

We passed an interesting open hay barn on the left, as lush greenery on both sides opened onto greener fields. Then we turned west on FM 3137 to take a look at Lake Palo Pinto, on a creek of the same name but—you guessed it—a tributary of that all-encompassing Brazos River! The 2,661-acre lake provides water sports and excellent fishing.

Returning to FM 4, we continued north through the

lovely, curving greenery and spectacular bluffs of the Palo Pinto Mountains. As we wound past cedar, mesquite, and pin oak, my husband remarked, "This is hillier than the Hill Country!" It certainly was a beautiful country road.

In Palo Pinto we took a look at the old jail and log cabin with their artifacts of area history. Then we passed the Palo Pinto Cemetery on the left as we turned east on U.S. 180 toward Mineral Wells. We were mystified by the hordes of modular buildings we saw in the middle of the countryside on our left, until we noticed the sign that read FEDERAL EMERGENCY MANAGEMENT AGENCY. Must be housing for emergencies, was our brilliant deduction, thinking of tornadoes and hurricanes.

Surrounded by the Palo Pinto Mountains, Mineral Wells was nationally famous in the late 19th century and even into the early 20th. It was the discovery of mineral waters that drew seekers searching for cures for a host of maladies. A historical marker marks the site of the Crazy Water Well, the first in the county; the belief back then was that the mineral waters could cure mental illness as well as other infirmities.

Another historical marker is on the spot of Edward P. Dismuke's water company, founded in 1913. His products included Dismuke's Pronto-lax, Dismuke's Eye Bath, and Dismuke's Famous Mineral Crystals. It's the only mineral water well operating today; the building has a drinking pavilion in addition to the well and bottling plant.

Lake Mineral Wells State Park encompasses 2,853 acres of post oak woodlands and grassy meadows set around Lake Mineral Wells. Wildlife in the large park includes white-tailed deer and wild turkeys. The relatively small lake is popular for swimming and fishing.

We returned to Fort Worth via the same FM 199 we'd started out on, after one last adventure: we headed north from Mineral Wells on U.S. 281 to follow the highway as it snaked through the Brazos Valley, giving us panoramic views of the valley floor as we mounted the bluffs above.

For More Information

Weatherford Chamber of Commerce, (817) 596-3801

Cleburne Chamber of Commerce, (817) 645-2455

Glen Rose Chamber of Commerce, (254) 897-2286

Dinosaur Valley State Park, (254) 897-4588

Granbury Chamber of Commerce, (940) 549-3355

Stephenville Chamber of Commerce, (254) 965-5313

Mineral Wells Chamber of Commerce, (817) 328-0850

12

North Texas to the Oklahoma Border and Small Towns with Famous Citizens

Getting there: From Dallas take I-35 north to McKinney, then State 5 through Melissa to State 121 to Bonham. From Bonham take U.S. 82 west through Ector to FM 2645 and turn north onto FM 1753 into Denison. From Denison go south on U.S. 75 to Sherman, west on State 56 to U.S. 82 to Gainesville, where the highway meets I-35, then south on FM 372 to FM 922 across the tip of Lake Ray Roberts to Tioga. From Tioga take U.S. 377 south to Pilot Point, then FM 455 to State 289 and into Dallas.

Highlights: Bonham, home of Sam Rayburn; Sherman and Lake Texoma; Denison, birthplace of President Eisenhower; Gainesville and the Frank Buck Zoo; Tioga, home of Gene Autry; Pilot Point and Bonnie and Clyde.

We headed north toward Oklahoma on I-35, leaving the interstate at the town of McKinney. Named for Collin McKinney, a signer of the Texas Declaration of Independence, this city of more than 30,000 has a lot of attractions to offer visitors.

First we drove around the town square admiring the courthouse, which is made of rough native stone with double windows outlined in red stone and a dark red–peaked roof with a clock tower perched atop it.

"Looks rather like a deep red dunce cap, doesn't it?" remarked my husband. I know he didn't mean to sound disparaging, and I had to agree with him, because it rather did. It rose to a point from all four angles. But then, the old-fashioned designs are what makes so many Texas county courthouses so attractive—until they decide to remodel them and in so doing, destroy so much of the charm. Luckily they haven't done this to McKinney's Collin County Courthouse— at least not yet.

Another building on the square was imposing, even though it's rather squeezed between Smith's Drugs and Dorothy's Cafe. It's the Greek-columned white marble First National Bank Building, with a golden eagle perched upon its roof and a historical marker under the portico.

Just south of the square on Chestnut Street we found several quaint Victorian and Greek Revival homes built between 1853 and 1910. They're furnished with period pieces, and are open for touring at certain times of the year.

The Old Post Office Museum is open only on Tuesday afternoons, but the handsome building, built in 1911 for $60,000, has walkways and peepholes used by the postal inspectors. The town's three museums are of varied interest. Bolin Wildlife Exhibit's eclectic displays range from mounted animal trophies from several states and foreign countries to memorabilia centered around a turn-of-the-century storefront.

The museum's Mobil Oil Company collection of a Model T circa 1913 and a Model A truck and roadster from 1928 were highlights of the transportation exhibits.

The Heard Natural Science Museum and Wildlife Sanctuary offers a collection of wildlife prints by Bessie Heard as an introduction to the 256-acre sanctuary. As for the Collin County Youth and Farm Museum, it's dedicated to preserving the county's agricultural heritage.

From McKinney, on State 5 we headed north toward the small town of Melissa, heading for Bonham. Crossing over the East Fork of the Trinity River, we passed Iron Kettle Antiques, housed in an attractive red barn with yellow trim, and it was tempting to stop and browse, but we decided to stay on course for Bonham. At Melissa we turned northeast on State 121, a straight, level road. Cattle (you can't get away from cattle in Texas) and creeks sped us on our way as we crossed Anna Creek, Loco Hill Creek, Sister Grove and Pilot Grove Creeks, through ranch and farmland, past sorghum fields (you can't get away from sorghum, either) and through small Trenton (pop. 690) to Bonham.

Speaker of the House Sam Rayburn put Bonham on the map, and the home of "Mr. Sam" in town is restored to 1961 elegance. The original furniture, china, and personal effects of Rayburn tell an interesting story of the man who served as speaker of the U.S. House of Representatives longer than any other person in American history.

The Sam Rayburn Library is an imposing white-porticoed building of Georgia marble. Inside the building, the library is an exact duplication of Speaker Rayburn's Washington office in the U.S. Capitol building. Details are precise, from the crystal chandelier hanging over the desk from the barrel-vaulted ceiling to the tile pattern on the floor. Among the fascinating mementos there we found a 2,500-year-old Grecian urn presented by the Athens Palace Guard in appreciation for American economic aid, and the many gavels used on historic occasions. The elegant deep red velvet drapes, patterned carpet, and photographs on the mantel, flanked by American and Texas flags behind the desk, add to an awesome still-felt presence of "Mr. Sam," whose portrait looked down on us from its spot over a maroon leather sofa.

Bonham is the seat of Fannin County and is situated on blackland prairie just south of the Red River, which marks the boundary between Texas and Oklahoma. The town is named for another hero of the Alamo, James Butler Bonham, and a statue honors him on the courthouse lawn. The Fannin County Museum, a repository of local history, is set in the town's restored 1900 Texas and Pacific Railroad Depot.

More rustic is Fort Inglish Park, with a replica of the log blockhouse and stockade built by Bailey Inglish in 1837. "Wouldn't that be fun to play in, if we were kids?" my companion remarked, and the replica is in such good condition it does look like something you might find at Six Flags in Frontier Town!

From Bonham we took State 78 north for about four miles to have a look at Lake Bonham. That 1,020-acre lake supplies the water for the whole city of Bonham as well as supplying the local folks with picnic sites, camping, and rest rooms.

We turned west on FM 898 toward FM 2645, a narrow road bordered by trees and shrubs and with more cattle in the fields beyond. We were on a Texas Lakes Trail whether we liked it or not—but we liked it, only leaving it behind when we came to FM 1753, which took us into Denison. That road curved around west when we thought we were going north, but it straightened out past the fields and farmhouses. We turned right, then left, and some goats eyed us as we went through Cherry Mound. ("There's the mound, where are the cherries?" complained my companion, whose favorite pie is cherry.)

We continued around the curves of the Texas Lakes Trail, turning left onto FM 120 and down a hill, around a curve, and into Denison.

Denison, of course, is famous as the birthplace of President Dwight D. Eisenhower. He may have grown up in Abilene, Kansas, but he was born here just five miles south of the Red River and the Oklahoma border. He was born on October 14, 1890, in a two-story white frame house at 208 E. Day Street. His father was a worker in the railway shops. The home was restored by the Eisenhower Birthplace Foundation and is open daily.

More exotic fame came to Denison with its grapes. Thomas Volney Munson arrived in Denison from Kentucky in 1876 and established a vineyard. When a plague of moths were destroying French vineyards, Munson sent over some hybrid varieties he had developed, varieties that were resistant to the particular moth in question. The French government was so grateful they bestowed the Legion of Honor on him. For all the world knows, all those fine French wines may very well come from descendants of those Texas grapes!

Munson's descendant, T. V. Munson of today's Munson's Vineyards, is known as the "World's Chief Vineyard Expert." A cutting off the family vine (all right, a chip off the old block!), Munson developed hybrid grape varieties that are on display on a five-acre plot of land on Grayson County College's campus, where a viticulture museum is in the works for the future.

The town of Denison started in 1872 when the Missouri, Kansas and Texas Railroad came down from the north, just a few years before Thomas Munson arrived. Now it's the gateway to Lake Texoma, a huge reservoir spreading over 89,000 acres of both Texas and Oklahoma. Formed, like most Texas lakes, by damming a river—this time the Red River—it's enjoyed jointly by both states, with both sides bragging that the fishing is the best in the nation. Denison Dam offers short, informative tours of the powerhouse, and there's an exhibit of the fossils that were unearthed during the construction.

Entertaining is the Grayson County Frontier Village, 13 authentic rustic buildings dating from 1840 to 1900, moved to the site and peopled by denizens of Denison in period costumes, doing whatever people used to do back then, like weaving, spinning, and blacksmithing. The village fronts on local Loy Lake, and the sunset over the lake was magnificent while we were there.

The old Traveler's Hotel in the E. M. Kohl Building on Main, circa 1893, took us by surprise with its tall peaked gables and almost-Tudor bay windows. It was being vigorously restored. "Maybe it'll be an interesting bed-and-breakfast place next time we come by," my husband said. It certainly looked like a perfect setting for just such an establishment.

Leaving Denison, we headed south on U.S. 75 to Sherman, which in its youth earned the title of "the Athens of Texas" because of the colleges and drama club—the epitome of gentility back in 1846, when the town was formed—that were started there. Today there's only Austin College left, chartered in 1849 in Huntsville but moved to Sherman in 1878.

The Red River Historical Museum in the town's old Carnegie Library has murals preserved since 1933. Pictures and artifacts tell the story of Grayson County, in which Denison is located. After submerging ourselves in history, we did some browsing in the antique shops around Lamar and Travis Streets, and then cruised over to Kelly Square for some shopping opportunities in the beautifully restored turn-of-the-century building containing boutiques and antiques.

Sherman was laid out a little to the west of its present location, but the scarcity of water and firewood forced a move to where it is today. "It's amazing that any town survived and grew, when you think of what life was like on the frontier," said my suddenly philosophical husband.

Subdued by such sober thoughts, we set out westward on State 56, meeting up with U.S. 82 at Whitesboro for awhile, driving toward Gainesville, a northern gateway to Texas at the crossroads of two major cross-country highways, U.S. 82 and I-35. While we could have taken U.S. 82 all the way, we thought perhaps a country road would be more interesting, so we took FM 56 paralleling 82 halfway, but there was nothing unusual along either stretch until we dropped south on FM 678, halfway between Whitesboro and Gainesville, entering Gainesville through the rolling hills of the Cross Timbers region.

Gainesville is another town that had a struggle with Indians "in the early days," as old-timers like to say, as though time didn't exist before then. It was a point on the California Trail and was settled in 1850, prudently near Fort Fitzhugh, an outpost that had been there since 1845. Even so, it was periodically raided by Indians until about 1868. But the town persisted, and once the Indian hostilities ceased, town fathers could concentrate on important matters like raising cattle and growing cotton.

The town is known for its brick-paved streets, lined with Victorian homes from the 19th century. With 26 noted, we found most of them on Denton, Church, and Lindsay Streets; the Chamber of Commerce was very helpful in identifying them.

We stopped by the Morton Museum of Cooke County, located in an old restored firehouse. (The present-day station and its big red fire engine are located at the back.) Museum exhibits cover a variety of displays, from geology and Indians to pioneer life.

The Frank Buck Zoo, named of course for the "bring 'em

back alive" adventurer Frank Buck, who happened to be a Gainesville native, is in Leonard Park just off I-35. The animals include flamingos, bears, zebras, camels, and an elephant, and although you shouldn't feed the animals, you can feed yourselves at shaded picnic tables.

We left Gainesville via FM 372 south through some more rolling hills of the Cross Timbers Region, passing panoramic views as we headed toward FM 922. The road led across the northern tip of Lake Ray Roberts, one of Texas's newest lakes. We could see the road curve up ahead of us as we went over a hill and then down into another curve. Even though the land along the road was fenced, signs warned drivers to be alert for cattle on the road.

Formed by damming the Elm Fork of the Trinity River, Lake Ray Roberts has a surface area of 29,350 acres. Parks are in the process of being developed, and at present there are two ramps for boat launchings. As the road led over low causeways with lake water on both sides, we wondered at the many dead tree trunks and branches sticking like pointed fingers out of the water. "Do you suppose the lake first floods and then kills them?" my companion asked, but I didn't have the answer. We'd seen the same thing crossing Lake Palestine in East Texas, but that isn't a new lake.

We turned east onto FM 922 into Tioga, population 625, a town that turned out to have a big surprise.

Tioga means "rushing waters"; it's the name of an Indian tribe back east in New York State. But for a while, it almost changed the name to Autry Springs. Back in 1936, singing cowboy and native son Gene Autry proposed the name change. He wasn't looking for an ego trip; evidently he planned to build a resort hotel and develop a spa around the mineral springs the town had back then.

Tioga Mineral Wells Company had been on the scene since 1886, and the company began to bottle and sell the water around 1902. The town's population swelled to more than a thousand, and the boom lasted until about 1936. But the wells sort of dried up, and Tioga was back to normal again.

As for the name change, seems like most of the town folk were for it, but one vote from one of the town's most influential citizens squashed it. Too bad, because Tioga was—and is—pretty proud of Autry's success.

Today Tioga has a new claim to fame. Seems that in 1989 *People Magazine* decided that Clark's Outpost Barbecue should be listed among the top 10 barbecue restaurants in America! We decided it was good, too!

If that wasn't enough excitement for one day, we headed south on U.S. 377 toward Pilot Point, about four times as large a town as Tioga. We'd heard that Bonnie and Clyde had robbed the bank there back in the 1930s, but nobody seemed to know exactly what the connection was. Part of the confusion could be caused by the fact that the movie *Bonnie and Clyde* was filmed on the site in 1967.

Pilot Point supposedly was named for a high point on the trail of covered wagons heading west, a landmark covered with a grove of trees, which made it a guidepost for the caravan's leader, or pilot. Now it's becoming an important quarter horse breeding center.

Full of romantic robberies and singing fame, we headed on back to Dallas by way of FM 455 east to State 289 and south to Dallas through the suburbs of Carrollton and Farmers Branch.

For More Information

McKinney Chamber of Commerce, (972) 542-0163

Bonham Area Chamber of Commerce, (903) 583-4811

Denison Chamber of Commerce, (903) 465-1551

Grayson County Frontier Village (Denison), (903) 463-2487

Sherman Chamber of Commerce, (903) 893-1184

Gainesville Chamber of Commerce, (940) 665-2831

Pilot Point Chamber of Commerce, (940) 686-5385

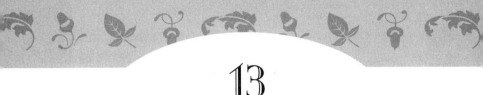

13

Cattle, Cars, Old Cemeteries, and Ducks

Getting there: From Austin take U.S. 183 south through Del Valle to FM 812 through Elroy and Red Rock. From Red Rock take a right on FM 20 to Lockhart. From Lockhart take FM 713 east through McMahan to State 304 north, then FM 535 north to State 95 and into Smithville, returning to Austin on State 71.

Highlights: McKinney Falls State Park; old cemeteries; fields of cattle; historical markers; Caldwell County Courthouse and Jail Museum; Lockhart's Clark Library; Central Texas Museum of Automotive History; Smithville's Railroad Historical Park and Museum; Buescher State Park.

Breezing south along U.S. 183, we stopped to take a look inside Callahan's General Store on the left side of the road. It's a real old-fashioned feed and ranch store, with chicks and ducks for sale as well as boots and saddles. Chicks, we could see; they become chickens—but ducks? Well, they were pretty cute, we decided, as we continued south.

When we saw the McKinney Falls sign, we turned right

onto McKinney Falls Parkway to see McKinney Falls State Park, which turned out to be a two-and-a-half-mile detour. A tall white tower on the left, with open, empty windows, caught our eye. The mystery was solved by the sign: CITY OF AUSTIN BILL ROBERTS FIRE TRAINING FACILITY. We were disappointed that there were no firefighters practicing; maybe another time?

We drove into the park all the way to the Upper McKinney Falls Scenic Overlook (the park ranger at the entrance gave us a map) and made a note of all the great camping facilities before returning to the parkway and taking Burleson Road as a shortcut back to 183.

Soon we crossed Cottonmouth Creek and turned left onto FM 812, a rather narrow two-lane road that winds past small frame houses and rows of mobile homes, either lived in or for sale. Although 183 had seemed to be out of the city, it took a little while on 812 until we felt we were out in the country. First we went past the City of Austin landfill on the left, and there were lots of old auto parts places on both sides. After a while we saw Salem Lutheran Church Cemetery on the left, which turned out to be the first of quite a number of old cemeteries we were to pass.

Finally the road left behind the remnants of the city and led out into open land, along flat, wire-fenced fields dotted with small cedars in almost perfect Christmas tree shapes. Beyond the cedars there were cattle, right and left. When I wondered at the number, my companion explained that, unlike dry West Texas, where it takes a lot of land to feed one animal, here the lush grassy fields, threaded with ponds and creeks, are able to support large herds. And large herds of every color cattle is what we saw, never just one or two lonesome cows.

Passing over South Fork Dry Creek (which wasn't dry), the road dipped down a small hill. A car appeared behind us, we pulled over to let it pass, and the occupants gave us a wave as they went on ahead. That was about all the traffic we were going to see on these country roads.

There was a Quickie Pickie convenience store and an old lawn mower junkyard on the left just before we entered Elroy. Immediately a sign pointed to a historical marker on the left, but we couldn't find it. We wheeled around and drove into the driveway of the Elroy Community Library and there it was on the door. The library was closed, but the plaque on the door said that Elroy had been settled in the 1890s by Swedish and German immigrants.

There not being much more to Elroy than that, we went on, surrounded by cattle and ponds with geese and duck. Crossing Maha Creek, the ranchland began to look more like farmland, with fields of sorghum or maybe cotton. As soon as we left Travis County and entered Bastrop County, we saw some cotton trailers on the right. They were empty, but little puffs of cotton clung to the wire-mesh sides. Then there began to be more gnarled oak patches, and even more duck ponds.

The flat land began to change to smoothly rolling small hills, and we laughed to see a smiling face painted high up on a tall white water tower on our left. Suddenly we saw a change from all the cattle: emus strutting around in a fenced area behind some low brush. "Some poor farmer stuck with them," my driver said. A few years ago, raising emus and marketing them as an alternative to beef had been touted as a good thing, but in this part of the world, at least, it hadn't amounted to much.

High View Ranch turned out to be a land development company, but the Angus cattle ranch just beyond really meant beef business with a BEEFMASTERS sign. And all along the road there were so many ponds with ducks, and even swans, that we began to understand why Callahan's General Store stocked ducks among the boots and saddles.

We drove across a small unnamed creek to see Old Red Rock Cemetery on the right, and then, just down the rolling

road, we came to the New Red Rock Cemetery. This was turning out to be a bonanza for folks interested in old cemeteries!
All the more since Red Rock appeared to the naked eye to
consist of nothing more than a large Shell station and the Red
Rock Storage Company, both at the intersection of FM 20.

We turned right onto 20 toward Lockhart, passing the first bit of cactus we'd seen so far. Past
Bateman Baptist Church was the Bateman
Cemetery, with picnic grounds and sheltered
tables across the road.

FM 80 was flat and wider, more open than
812, with wider vistas on both sides of the road. The
minute we passed the sign announcing that we were entering
Caldwell County, railroad tracks joined us along the right side
of the road, and we could smell oil in the air. Sure enough, we
passed a yardful of unused pump jacks identified by a sign:
TRINIDAD PETROLEUM COMPANY. Then suddenly we were surrounded by working pump jacks pumping away in the fields
and all among the trees.

Then the road became nice and rolling, with a sign marking it as a Texas Independence Trail. Soon we came to another
historical marker, this one commemorating both the Lincecom Cemetery, 1847 (the marker stated that Lincecom, cre-
ator of Caldwell County, was a cousin of James Bowie) and
Isham Jones Good, died 1835, who fought in the Texas War of
Independence, escaping the infamous Goliad Massacre. He
was the first sheriff of Caldwell County.

On the way into Lockhart through open vistas and rolling
land, we came to yet another cemetery, Brite Cemetery, and
into town. We were ready for some of that great Lockhart
barbecue, either at Black's ("The oldest BBQ house in Texas
continuously owned by the same family, since 1932") or the
Chisholm Trail Bar-B-Que on the opposite end of downtown.
Sharing beef at one and ribs at the other, we pronounced then
both excellent.

Big-town Lockhart (pop. 9,000+) was originally named Plum Creek, and it was the site of a fierce battle with Comanches in 1840. Took a bunch of settlers and Texas Rangers to win the Battle of Plum Creek—and then the town was renamed for pioneer surveyor Byrd Lockhart. There's a historical marker in Lockhart City Park commemorating the battle, even though it didn't actually take place right in town.

For years the Comanches had the advantage over first the Spanish/Mexicans and later the Anglo settlers (after the Texas War of Independence) because they could let loose a hail of arrows while the defenders were busy reloading their one-shot-at-a-time guns. What changed all that was Sam Colt's invention, the Colt revolver. The Comanches couldn't hold out against guns that kept on firing. In the 1870s the city was the southern end of the Chisholm Trail, and there's an enactment of the battle every June during the Chisholm Trail Roundup.

The Dr. Eugene Clark Library is something to see: not only is it the oldest continuously used library in Texas, it was modeled after the Villa Rotunda in Vicenza, Italy, with gorgeous stained-glass windows. Caldwell County Courthouse in the middle of the square is unusual, too, with cupolas, turrets, and other fancy embellishments of the 1890s, when it was built. The Caldwell County Jail Museum is a sort of red-brick Norman castle keep. Cells now contain exhibits from pioneer homes, as well as early farming implements.

Leaving Lockhart, we backtracked on 20 for about four miles to FM 713 and McMahan, past farms and ranchland, farm houses, and occasional groves of oak trees. We saw a small windmill on the left and some cactus before we came to yet another cemetery, or rather, two: Flemmings Cemetery and Jeffrey Cemetery. Both were to the right, around Bethel Primitive Baptist Church, dated 1852.

Turning on to FM 304, we headed north past FM 535, the road to Rosanky, because although the address of the Central Texas Museum of Automotive History is listed as Rosanky, it turned out not to be in that little town after all. Nope, it's on 304, about two and a half miles north of 535.

The museum is dedicated to the preservation of historic automobiles, accessories, and such, tracing the development from high wheelers and steam buggies of the turn of the century to the aerodynamic sports and passenger cars of today. You can imagine what a sight this was, with anywhere from 100 to 115 vehicles on display. (An additional 50 wait in the wings on a rotational basis.)

Early European estate cars, town cars, limousines, sports cars—what a display they make, along with gasoline and oil pumps, oil company signs, license plates from around the world, all spit and polished to perfection.

Leaving the museum, we drove the two and a half miles back to FM 535 and turned left past cedar and oak woods, more cattle and duck ponds, and even another emu farm. Tiny String Prairie consisted of a house, fire department, and community center along the road, although of course there were other houses scattered along the road and over the flat fields in the distance.

A bunch of cows in a field were munching on a hay mound as we came to Rosanky. A Diamond Shamrock Quick Stop was on our left as we crossed some railroad tracks, and the tracks turned and followed us along the road. Took maybe a minute to go through Rosanky, and just out of town we overtook a pickup truck loaded with hay.

"Do you realize, except for Lockhart, this is the only traffic the entire day, except for the car with the people who waved at us as we let it pass way back around Elroy?" we both exclaimed at once. Talk about relaxing driving! We cruised along, enjoying the dense oak woods, laced with red pyracantha berries, on each side of the narrow road. No traffic, no billboards, just country farmland (one place had named itself Duck Crossing), and lots of oak forest.

We almost hated for it to end as we cruised around a curve and down a hill onto Highway 95. Left was Smithville, a delightful small town (pop. 3,000+) with its historic Main Street lined with antique shops. Smithville is another of Texas's railroad towns now full of historic memorabilia since the trains left. Main Street ends at the Railroad Historical Park and Museum featuring both Union Pacific and Katy (MKT) cabooses. In fact, back in the 1800s the town moved from another location in order to get in on the new rail line.

The museum is in a Katy depot built from materials salvaged from a former 1890s station, and across the street you'll find good home-cooked food at The Courtyard Restaurant. The Back Door Cafe, back on Main Street among the antiques, is another local place to eat, with a buffet on Sundays. The Smithville Heritage Society has a museum in an old house on Main. Another historical home is the Burleson House, named for the man who once owned a great deal of the land hereabouts.

Large and popular Buescher State Park is nearby, close to the famous "Lost Pines of Texas." They're not really lost, it's just that nobody knows why they're here when all other related pines are far away in the Piney Woods of East Texas. Nevertheless, the 1,730 acres of scenic, rolling parkland are a plus for Smithville. The usual fine camping, shelters, picnicking, fishing (on Lake Buescher), hiking, and nature study opportunities are here for the taking.

For More Information

Callahan's General Store, (512) 385-3452

McKinney Falls State Park, (512) 389-8900

Lockhart Chamber of Commerce, (512) 398-2818

Black's Barbecue, (512) 398-2712

Chisholm Trail Bar-B-Que, (512) 398-6027

Smithville Chamber of Commerce, (512) 237-2313

Central Texas Museum of Automotive History, (512) 237-2635

The Courtyard Restaurant, (512) 237-5314

Back Door Cafe, (512) 237-3128

Buescher State Park, (512) 237-2241

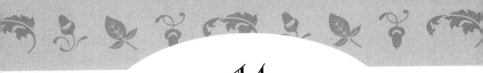

14

Central Texas and the Brazos River

Getting there: From Temple take Loop 363 east to FM 438, then FM 935 to State 7 to Marlin. Take State 6 south to Business 6 and FM 712 to the Brazos River. Then FM 413 to Rosebud and down U.S. 77 to Cameron; west on State 36 to FM 2268 to Salado. You'll return to Temple on I-35.

Highlights: Marlin; historic hot springs; Brazos River and Falls on the Brazos River Park; historical markers; Cameron's Magnolia House and the Ports to Plains Highway, connecting Texas heartland to coastal ports; Salado on Salado Creek.

Although we'd left the city behind, there was plenty of traffic around us along Loop 363 for quite a ways. Finally the loop divided, east and west, and we went east over railroad tracks loaded with tank cars and around curves past fenced land full of cattle on the right. The road rose between high green banks and went down a small hill under the overpass to Little Flock Road. We passed lots of parked farm machinery, big wet ponds, and clumps of oak trees.

It was funny to see a lone little bright red Volkswagen Beetle parked way in the middle of a field on our right. Next we passed Harvest Baptist Church on one side and a stone quarry on the other side of the intersection of FM 438.

Turning right on 438, we bumped along on a very narrow road between bright green fields on both sides. As we passed the Cen-Tex Nursery sign, we came upon a whole group of fallen-down buildings, weatherbeaten and picturesque, the kind that make artistic black-and-white photographs.

Then there was a lot of farm machinery jumbled together on the left as the road curved past very muddy Cottonwood Creek Road. Far away across the fields beyond that, a large old-fashioned farmhouse loomed up majestically in the distance.

An oncoming truck passed us, the only other vehicle we saw since we left Loop 313 behind us. "The land looks well kept, but not the houses," observed my chauffeur as we veered left past Apple Cider Road, and the road became flat and curved. As we ended a wide curve along what had become a very zigzag road, a trim red barn put the lie to his words. Next we passed through the small settlement of Cenaville, where our road took a sharp left turn past a Shell station. (We would have found ourselves on FM 3369 if we hadn't been alert, and heaven knew where *that* went.)

A pile of old refrigerators was dumped in a field on the right, and past a feedmill and Bottoms East Road, the tall pale green tower of the Superior Public Water System rose up into the sky. "Look at that pretty yellow house on the right," I said. "Why does that other one have bricks scattered all over the roof?"

"To maybe hold tar paper down?" was the question that answered my question as we passed a duck pond and a windmill. Then the road dead-ended onto FM 935 at tiny Belfalls. We turned east, and there was a sign telling us NOW ENTERING

FALLS COUNTY. Belfalls Cemetery was on the right, next to a drainage ditch. Now there were few trees; it was all open farmland, and an even bumpier road.

We passed several more ruined buildings on the left, and then along came a nice-looking modern farmhouse, along with the usual cattle and pond. Past the sign to Durango Road on the right, we saw a triangular pen absolutely crammed with cattle. "Waiting for market?" we wondered. As we passed the sign to the Union Cemetery on the left, the road still curving and bumpy, we spied a whole spread of tidy matching buildings—house, barn, outbuildings—set in wide green fields with lots of cattle. On a tall flagpole in front of the house, Old Glory waved brightly in the breeze.

Two more cars passed us at once, and then we saw what looked like small rodeo grounds on the left, with barrels (for barrel racing) and a guy riding a horse.

"Do you think it's a practice place?" we asked each other as we went on to see, all at once, the Carolina Cemetery sign, Deer Haven Farm, and a forest of oak trees, all on our left. We zoomed past Little Deer Creek Baptist Church as we crossed the intersection of U.S. 77. The church was as quaint as its name, clean and white, with a tall white steeple pointing into the blue sky.

Cattle, cattle everywhere, fields of them left and right as we crossed over a narrow bridge with bright yellow posts over some anonymous (no identifying sign) water. Although we knew we weren't in oil country, there were big oil tanks on the right. Big trees, too, sort of a small forest, but the ground between the trees was covered with piles of fallen branches.

Ah, a change from the cattle—a whole field of goats to our left as we turned right onto State 7 for the seven miles into Marlin. We laughed at the big blue sign in the middle of a field. Huge white letters were painted on it, proclaiming FOR SALE YOUNG PAIRS. Pairs of what? Goats? Children?

As we came to a bridge over the Brazos River, we read an EAT MORE BEEF sign as the road became wider and smoother, lined with quite a few more picturesque ramshackle buildings. The river originally was named Brazos de Dios, Spanish for "Arms of God," possibly because when the Coronado expedition back in Spanish times got lost and were almost dying of thirst, they fell into the river and named it thus in thankfulness.

Cruising past a ready-mix cement plant on the left, we came into Marlin.

Marlin was established in the 1830s, and the early settlers faced a lot of attacks by the Indians. Sites of these conflicts are marked around town, but most of Marlin's glory came from a hot artesian well. (History remarks that the settlers often came in second best in those conflicts.)

Drillers in the early 1890s struck water, and its purported curative qualities turned Marlin into a spa that attracted thousands who came to bathe in the healthful waters.

It's all gone today, although the town is investigating ways of using geothermal energy, and the chamber of commerce and the hospital are heated by hot spring water. But you might want to stop for antiques: there's an antique store immediately to the right on State 7 as you swing into town, and several more on the main street.

From Marlin we took State 6 south, turning right when we saw the Falls Park sign. The road curved past Peaceful Rest Memorial Park on the right, and we drove along looking for signs of the park. Sure enough, along came a sign for FM 712, three miles to the Park.

Turning left, we soon came to a historical marker, so we stopped and read: "Site of Bucksnort, settled in 1837 by members of Marlin and Menefee families. The name was coined by a drunk patron of the saloon, but by the 1850s Bucksnort was no longer a viable community."

"Translation: Everybody gone," said my driver as we curved under a railroad overpass, driving carefully through a large puddle of water. The roadside sign read LOW WATER CROSSING, with a flood gauge leaning rather tiredly against the cement wall of the overpass. Next we were surprised to see on our left quite a complex of big blocks of gray cement buildings. There was nobody else on the road, so we slowed down and backed up to read the sign: THE WILLIAM P. HOBBY CORRECTIONAL INSTITUTE. The institute buildings were spread out all over the flat fields—and not too close to the road. Strung out along the road across from the place was a row of NO PARKING ON ROAD signs. We figured they didn't want anyone waiting to aid in any quick getaways!

Not too much farther on, we came to a sign and a gravel road leading into Falls on the Brazos River Park. The river was nice and wide, but the falls were a disappointment; they were more like a long low dam stretched across the river. But they evidently appeared more impressive to the couple we saw at the river's edge: the woman was busy videotaping the scene.

But what with the camping and picnic spots lining the river, it looked like a relaxing place to come back to for a picnic and some fishing. There was a children's playground, too, and a concession stand.

Leaving the park, we turned back on 712. Instead of warning "low water crossing," the sign on this side of the underpass said WATCH FOR WATER ON ROAD, and we did, driving slowly as we noticed that the gauge on this side was registering about six inches of water.

Back on Business 6, we turned left to Rosebud and came to a bonus: not one, but two historical markers side by side. The first one was to General Thomas Harrison. As a veteran of the Mexican war and in defense of the Texas frontier, he was wounded three times. Moreover, he had his horse shot from under him five times. Guess he really earned his future office, of district judge, in 1866.

Next to this was marked the site of colonial capital, Sarahville de Viesa, founded in 1834 by Sterling Robertson. He named the town for both his mother and for Augustin de Viesa, governor of the Province of Coahuila and Texas. (Texas was part of Mexico then.) The town, target of Indian hostilities, was abandoned in 1836.

Next we coasted past Fall County Fence Builders, with huge piles of cedar logs in front. (The *Texas Almanac* says that cedar posts are part of the county's farm income.) With Washington Cemetery on the right, we found Highway 6 flat, straight, and smooth. We caught up with some traffic, too, but not too much. We got a laugh out of the red barn on the right with "Gig Em Aggies" painted very large on the side. (The Aggies are Texas A&M students, rivals of the University of Texas, whom they call "Tea Sippers.")

As we veered east onto FM 413 through tiny Highbank, a sleek black-and-tan dog ran out of a house yard and chased our car. On the other side, a pretty blue house had a porchful of chairs but nobody was sitting in them. A bunch of cattle were busily feeding at a mound of hay, and then we passed more derelict barns and more cattle.

The road crossed over the Brazos River again, and a big Brahmin cow stared at me, looked me right in the eye, as we cruised on toward Rosebud. Next were two large house trailers planted solidly in a grove of trees, while a blue jeep zoomed by us. FM 413 joined FM 2027 where a field of goats faced a gas station/corner store. Shaggy cattle were lying down in the fields, and there were horses, too, and just before we coasted into Rosebud we passed three very dilapidated silos and a barn.

But Rosebud seemed to be a pretty little town. The narrow road went right through town, past rows of tidy little houses. Then suddenly we were at the intersection of U.S. 77 and on to Cameron.

A small town in the rich agricultural area of Milam County, Cameron was settled in the 1840s by a mixed group of pioneers—Spanish, Czech, and German among them. The town was named for Ewen Cameron, a Scots Highlander who fought in the Texas Revolution. The county is named for another freedom fighter, Ben Milam, whose statue you can see on the grounds of the courthouse.

The Magnolia House, built in 1895 with every piece of wood chosen for rarity and beauty of grain, encouraged the Texas Historical Commission to say, cautiously, that it "may be the finest home of its size and type in the country." It's authentically furnished, too.

The Milam County Historical Museum is housed in a restored county jail. We always like to take a look at the cells, shackles, and gallows tower in these old jailhouses of the 1890s. Now the cells are filled with frontier memorabilia.

From Cameron we took State 36, a segment of the Ports to Plains Highway, which connects the Texas heartland to the coastal ports. Heading west, we passed Shorty's Fruit & Vegetable Stand before the road became rolling again, lined with oak trees and lots of underbrush. We found some traffic on this important road, and we didn't mind in the least when the big white pickup truck in front of us pulled into the big VFW Post on the left.

The road went through Buckholts (pop. 325) to FM 437, and we knew we were in cotton, as well as sorghum, country, when we read the big sign on the right saying BUY GROWN AND MADE IN USA COTTON PRODUCTS. As we rolled under a railroad bridge, the next sign told us we were "entering Bell County" again.

Seemed like the country roads we were on zigzagged in and out of three counties: Bell, Falls, and Milam. According to the *Texas Almanac*, all three are rich agricultural areas, with income from cattle, goats, sheep, turkeys, and hogs, although all we saw were lots of cattle and a smattering of goats. But we did see lots of sorghum, cotton, and hay fields—and lots of hay!

Next came the town of Rogers, with its sign proclaiming WELCOME TO ROGERS: GOOD SCHOOLS, GOOD CHURCHES, GOOD PEOPLE. We noticed that the Rogers Eagles football team had a banquet coming up. We turned south onto FM 2268, and the road became bumpy again. Then we were in more rolling country, with cattle and big ponds as we entered Milam County. Driving across the bridge over Little Brazos River, we noticed people fishing below on the river banks.

A man on a tractor at the edge of the road waved as we caught sight of a red barn, which would have been hard to miss. It had a big Lone Star of Texas flag painted on its side. Next we turned right onto FM 2268 toward Holland, around a big, wide curve where a white building and tall white steeple welcomed passersby to the Val Verde Baptist Church and cemetery.

"Look at that old water well on the left," exclaimed my driver, but drat! I missed it. But I did see a bunch of hay bales all in a long row, each bale dressed up in a covering of white plastic. As we passed the sign to Rosanky Road, we saw a white tank painted with a big red-and-pink heart. There was a big Brahmin cattle spread on the right past another big pond and some oak woods.

Then the road jogged onto State 95 into Holland (pop. 1,118). There we had to quick turn left past a Fina Station to continue following 2268 west. The tall water tower on the left touted the Holland Hornets as we turned left to follow the road 11 miles to Salado.

Salado's Stagecoach Inn is famous for its past as a busy stop on the Chisholm Trail back in the 19th century (although it was called the Shady Villa Inn back then). Historical figures such as General George Custer, Jesse James, and Robert E. Lee tarried here. Today the old frame building is a fine restaurant; the lodging part's taken care of by the surrounding and very modern motor inn.

Salado is named for its creek—*salado* means "salty" in Spanish—and the creek was Texas's first designated natural landmark. Today's Pace Park along the creek was an Indian campsite way back before recorded time, and it makes a lovely picnic spot.

Incorporated in 1867, the town prospered when it was the home of Salado College, but when the railroad passed it by, the college closed and so sort of did the town. But there are 18 historic sites listed on the National Register of Historic Homes. And nowadays it's the home of several notable artists and craftspeople, so we took time to see some galleries, antique shops, and women's fashion shops before we drove onto I-35 and back to Temple.

For More Information

Marlin Chamber of Commerce, (817) 883-2171

Cameron Chamber of Commerce, (817) 697-4979

Magnolia House (Cameron), (817) 697-4395

Salado Chamber of Commerce, (254) 947-5040

Stagecoach Inn (Salado), (254) 947-5111

Index